Eye movements, surprise reactions and cognitive development

Modern approaches to the diagnosis and instruction of multi-handicapped children

13

Eye movements, surprise reactions and cognitive development

K. M. Wilton
*Lecturer in Education, University of
Canterbury, New Zealand*

and

F. J. Boersma
*Professor of Educational Psychology, University of
Alberta, Canada*

With an introduction by
H. Mackworth
*Professor of Psychology and Psychiatry,
Stanford University*

1974
Rotterdam University Press

Acknowledgment*

The authors wish to acknowledge the National Research Council of Canada (NRC Operating Grant APA270) and the Donner Canadian Foundation whose funds financed this investigation. A special word of thanks is also due to Richard Barham, Gerry Kysela and Tom Maguire for their constructive comments, to Patricia Fleming for her assistance in data collection, and to the Edmonton Public School Board for their co-operation. Order of authorship was determined by flipping a coin.

* This monograph was written while the second author was a visiting professor at the Free University of Amsterdam, the Netherlands (Psychological Research Laboratory).

Contents

Introduction

I have had the good fortune to be concerned with the invention of various eye-camera procedures; these have been devised to indicate where people are looking in order to try to understand how they think. By far the most rewarding aspects of this activity has been that these cameras have introduced me to a wide range of scientific friends. These are all pioneers who have been quick to cross national borders (and sometimes even the boundaries between scientific disciplines) to make use of these devices or compare ideas and data. These friends have come from a dozen different countries: Japan, Sweden, France, Canada, Austria, Australia, USSR, England, Holland, Iran, New Zealand, and the United States. Cognitive studies on the line of sight are fairly recent, but they have a long history dating back almost a century to the famous observations by Prof. Javal (1878). It was in 1878 that Javal looked directly at the eyes of school children in Paris and found that they moved along the lines of print in jumps and pauses (Lévy-Schoen, 1969). Perhaps then it would be doubly appropriate for the forth coming XXIst. International Congress of Psychology to celebrate that Centenary since this meeting is to be held in France in the very same city that these simple and important observations were taken so long ago. To this day, Paris remains the city where some of the most incisive uses of the line-of-sight approach are being made by Vurpillot (1968, 1972) and her remarkable research group.

Equally effective is the group centered around Boersma in the University of Alberta at Edmonton in Canada. It was the Canadian psychologist, especially those in this highly productive laboratory, who were among the first to realize the potential uses of these line-of-sight methods. I therefore find it an honor as well as a pleasure to be invited to make a few comments to introduce this volume by Wilton and Boersma. Clearly this is the first of a series of volumes on a range of investigations undertaken at Edmonton over many years.

The present book appears at a time in which Canadian psychology is just starting to receive some hard-won recognition for its achievements

1

since World War II. The most recent tribute came from the United States when in 1973 the American Psychological Association went to Canada for the first annual meeting ever to be held outside the US borders. This was an historic gathering in Montreal, attended by 20,000 people. Perhaps I can best indicate the approaches and achievements of Wilton and Boersma by placing their thinking against the background of ideas I obtained by listening to a few of the many distinguished speakers at this Montreal meeting. In this manner, I hope to illustrate how this volume is not only important for the evidence and concepts it considers directly. It is also of significance in another way. Being at the forefront of research, the authors indicate certain working assumptions now being adopted by an increasing number of investigators in the area of cognitive psychology, those who are looking at the basic aspects, and also those who are considering the more practical aspects of this subject which has grown up in the last decade.

Value of experimental studies of individuals

At the Montreal meeting, for instance, one of the leading Canadian psychologists, Professor Donald Hebb, spelled out some of the working assumptions that have been so successfully put to the test in the present volume. He emphasized that the central concern of psychology should be about man's mind and thought. But he strongly rejected the flamboyant, fast and inaccurate introspective method in favor of the slow-but-sure experimental approach. No one with Hebb's background of research achievement would underestimate the importance of sound speculation as a preliminary stage in most experimental studies. Basically his line of argument here was that some of the most important speculations on the nature of the mind and its mechanisms were likely to come from physiological psychology. Similarly, the present authors have based a great deal of their work on Sokolovian ideas on the physiological basis of perception. Professor Hebb was also characteristically eclectic in welcoming the valuable European-style approaches to psychology exhibited by Piaget and the Geneva school for their insightful use of direct observational methods. Clearly, the reliance on the Piaget fund of ideas by the present authors needs no emphasis here, since they obviously have made important contributions towards some of these concepts started by Piaget.

The research benefits of experience in the clinic and classroom

A further basic assumption shared by the present authors and Hebb was that he underscored the Claude Bernard view that those who bring a good theoretical background to the classroom or the clinic can often come up with some novel ideas. This view was also adopted by Professor J.J. Jenkins of the University of Minnesota during his presidential address to the Division of Experimental Psychology at the 1973 APA Conference. Here Professor Jenkins specifically noted the value of including clinical experience in the formulation of problems for subsequent laboratory study by experimental methods. Professor Jenkins, one of the leading psycholinguists in the United States, suggested that the most important problem to be studied in psychology was the interaction between the experience an individual brings into an experimental room and the stimuli within the particular experimental task with which he is confronted. This idea of the effects of the context that the subject brings to the stimuli is basic to the research by Wilton and Boersma. They are analysing these interactions in situations which involve some of the simplest ways that people transform or translate the input stimuli.

PRACTICAL IMPLICATIONS FOR MEDICAL AND EDUCATIONAL CARE IN LEARNING DISABILITIES

Next, we turn to the ways in which these investigations by Wilton and Boersma can give really practical benefits to both the classroom and the clinic. The Montreal meeting had an interesting symposium on the overlapping worlds between learning disabilities and mental retardation. I believe that it is in these realms that the greatest practical benefits will come, by extending this present type of research. Not all the procedures will necessarily involve eye-camera methods; but appropriately enough, the eye-camera methods in Edmonton have clearly struck oil. But nobody suggests that the procedures used to find oil are always the best to refine it. The new ideas found will lead on the new educational and diagnostic tasks. I suggest that quite often eye-camera approaches can indicate simpler slide-projection tasks in which required data can be obtained in more convenient ways, especially when time is as short as it is in many classrooms or clinics.

Better diagnostic classification for learning disabilities

It was Wedell (1973) who made the key remark about learning disabilities. Anyone who is trying to help a child with a learning disability has to know as much as possible about the pattern of his strengths and weaknesses. At

3

the Montreal meeting, two other authorities on learning disabilities, Professor Helmer Myklebust of the University of Illinois and Professor John Niesworth of Pennsylvania State University, agreed on a number of points. For instance, they agreed on the remarkable state of confusion that exists in the classification of learning disabilities. Never in the history of human conditions have so many entirely different disorders been lumped under one inclusieve term. Secondly, they agreed that the best way out of this diagnostic jungle was to follow the approach of getting to know the individual child more thoroughly, especially by individual one-to-one studies of his strengths and weaknesses on a range of performance tests.

This emphasis on the value of the individual test approach is particularly important at a time when there is a complete breakdown of the group testing programs based on pencil-and-paper testing. Absolutely no scientific authorities now believe that group pencil-and-paper testing can diagnose the strengths and weaknesses of individual children as regards the full range of their various skills in processing information. For example, despite huge advertising claims, there is no possibility, either now or on the horizon, of learning the skills profile of children entering school from the pencil-and-paper group tests termed reading readiness tests. The sub-test data of such tests do *not* give and are not meant to give these data. Some day such group tests may be swept away. It is therefore important to distinguish between the group and the one-to-one individual tests. Many authorities, of whom Myklebust (1973) is the most outstanding, have hard scientific evidence that the distinction is valid. The fact is that person-to-person skill testing *is* effective; this is therefore quite different from group pencil-and-paper testing which is usually done for administrative purposes rather than to benefit the individual. The important point here is that the one-to-one test situation can provide measurements of the various skills possessed by the learning disabled child that are of the utmost importance to him and to children like him.

Need for improved diagnosis for children with learning disabilities

Suppose we spend some more time looking at the existing diagnostic confusion in detail because it does indicate why we need new methods and insights such as we can get from eye-camera studies of the Wilton and Boersma type. The plain fact is that it is exceedingly difficult to assess the skills of a child who is so lacking in language abilities as to be almost non-verbal. Strong evidence in support of this view came recently from a study by Rosenthal, Eisenson and Luckau (1972) at the Stanford University School of Medicine.

4

These researchers examined 82 children in terms of 32 different aspects of either test performance scores or case histories. The best available highly detailed procedures were used to gather test scores, clinical evidence, and brain recordings of the customary EEG type. The children had arrived at the hospital clinic with a wide range of different diagnostic labels. The data were then entered into a computer for an impartial analysis to see if children could be appropriately grouped under a priori label. The study showed in brief that they generally could not. Only two clusters of children could be seen. The first cluster was somewhat of a surprise in itself because it lumped together 'mentally retarded' with 'autistic' children. But the second cluster was even more surprising: it showed that it was impossible to distinguish between an even wider range of diagnostic labels. The second cluster showed that current practice cannot tell one condition from another when the children coming into the clinic arrive with labels like 'late developer', 'severe hearing loss', 'neurologically handicapped', 'aphasic child with speech comprehension difficulties', etc. Obviously it is not too hard to determine hearing losses, but these may well have further effects on the ability to process information. This brings up the more general fact that any given child may well be suffering from two or more of the conditions that can cause a learning disability.

For administrative purposes it is usually necessary to label handicapped children with some such label as 'children with learning disabilities' or as 'educationally handicapped children'. Perhaps an even more neutral term such as 'special education children' might be even better. But at least the above terms do not have the ego-destroying effects of mindlessly labelling children with high-sounding terms such as 'minimal brain damage', 'neurological impairment', 'minimal brain injury' or 'brain dysfunction', or 'dyslexic case'. Another way in which such labels can do harm is to delay the day when the appropriate remedial experience is made available to the child.

Better educational methods to remedy learning disabilities

Estes (1970) has recently surveyed the relationships between learning theory and mental development. He mentions, for instance, that a strong implication of the Zeaman and House (1963) views on the role of attention in visual discrimination by mentally retarded children is that the training and education of such children should concentrate heavily on ways of modifying attention to the relevant cues in the various situations they are most likely to encounter.

In their conclusions (Chapter 4), the authors of the present study made

5

the point that eye-movement behavior reflects differential cognitive activity in mentally retarded persons. This has been found in a number of studies by the Boersma group. Perhaps the greatest immediate research need is to understand the conditions under which it is, or is not, an advantage to the mentally retarded to have repeated verbal instructions on the most relevant cues to be inspected in the given visual task. The eye-camera procedures make it immediately clear to the investigator whether the instructions are being followed, and even simple shaping procedures can be adopted to guide the gaze from resting on the part of the scene that is fairly helpful onto the most informative area of all. Clearly, the advice or directions should sometimes be non-verbal, as for example, when children are perhaps very deaf or totally without linguistic skills. In this case, it is useful quite literally to point out where to look.

In regard to children who are able to understand speech fairly well, a most important recent discovery has been made by Roger Cooper (1974) working in the Department of Psychology at Stanford University. He has found that when normal adults look at a matrix of line drawings, they will pick out with their gaze the one picture which corresponds to the spoken word they are hearing at that moment from an on-going tape-recorded story. It is obvious that a procedure like this should be useful not only in the assessment of the audio-to-pictorial transformations that the child can undertake, but it might also be valuable as a training method to improve the abilities of mentally retarded and language disabled children to achieve a higher level of skill in this kind of situation. If directed looking works well as a training method, we must find out which practice situations transfer most easily to real word tasks.

Professor Niesworth (at the Montreal meeting on learning disabilities) emphasized that milder levels of disability were the harder conditions to distinguish from each other. Wedell (1973) notes that the repeated testing of a child during a series of learning experiences is often a revealing procedure. This idea of diagnostic teaching could well be tried in cases of mild learning disability since, for instance, the eye-camera measures and other test scores may show a different pattern of improvement or non-improvement in the different disabilities.

Imagery and its role in information processing

The highly paradoxical situation about learning disabilities and mental retardation is that many practical problems related to diagnosis and teaching of such disorders simply cannot be solved until there have been more basic investigations like those of Wilton and Boersma. One central question is to discover the extent to which children and adults have two alternative pathways from their environment to their stored experience. Paivio (1971) has, for instance, favored this idea of two distinct systems: one for the pictorial images and the other for verbal materials. Bower (1972) and Sheehan (1973) have much evidence on the role of imagery in the processing of information. The functions of internal representations and mental models have recently become respectable, and indeed essential ingredients in the mix of scientific problems with high priority. No longer are the questions of imagery to be regarded as a bunch of far-out wild ideas best left to the lunatic fringe of scientific society.

The main concept is that pictorial items providing information on spatially organized objects and events are dealt with by the visual imagery system, whereas items involving words are processed by the verbal system. The developmental aspects of this double system involve the question as to how children normally learn to extrapolate from the immediate stimulus situation. Most authorities agree that transformation of the stimulus input is achieved by the age of about 7 years in normal children, as in the conservation tasks discussed by Wilton and Boersma in the present volume. But Bruner (1964) disagrees with Piaget and Inhelder (1971) on exactly how this is done. Bruner (1964) takes the view that the verbal system is sufficiently well-developed to take over from the iconic pictorial processing system by the age of 7. But Piaget and his group (1970) favor the idea that this is done by non-verbal anticipatory images. Paivio (1970) thinks that both viewpoints are correct and suggests that at this age there are developments in both systems.

Pribram (1971) has discussed a similar distinction between perceptual images and images of achievement processing systems. He considers that the images of achievement contain all the input and outcome information necessary for the next step of that achievement. Such patterns of motor activity include the verbal motor programs of speech production and recognition (Liberman, Shankweiler, and Studdert-Kennedy, 1967), and their study is therefore important for the treatment of children who are linguistically retarded or who are suffering from other learning disabilities. It is therefore of considerable interest to learn anything we can about the links between imagery and the formation of a new plan of action.

The role of achievement images in anticipatory processes

Wilton and Boersma give some good clues for the study of these problems, which should be of interest to academic and clinician alike. I must therefore mention some of the highlights in their fact-filled volume. Outstandingly interesting is their direct evidence from line-of-sight recording that *normal children* who were good at transforming stimuli were much more active in visually searching the display than those who were not. The good transformers, (able to conserve in Piagetian tasks) looked back and forth between the two paired displays *twice* as often as the other normal children who were unable to transform stimuli. Moreover, the *mentally retarded* group showed no such effect. Perhaps the mentally retarded group found it harder to develop anticipatory images because they could not even store quite briefly the stimulus patterns in perceptual image form. Certainly Osaka (1972) of Kyoto University and Bryant (1972) of Oxford University have evidence consistent with this idea, for children and adults respectively.

Important differences were found between the normals and the retarded children on another simple line-of-sight measure. This measure was the time spent on either of the two alternative items during their judgment, especially the ratio of time which was obtained by counting the number of motion picture frames showing the gaze resting on either of the two items. On this examination-time measure, the *normal children* who were good at transforming stimuli were found to give about equal time to the two items on display, ratio of 1 : 1. But the normal children who were poor stimulus transformers spent 65 per cent more time looking at what they judged to be the greater of the two items on display, a ratio of 1.6:1. This is important because it is entirely objective data which further confirms Piaget's idea that one of the simplest and best measures of perceptual and cognitive development is the extent to which the child can ignore salient cues to discover less salient but more significant stimuli. With the eye-camera, the child can be studied directly to determine the extent to which he can literally look past the eye-catching stimuli for the important stimuli; this is the famous 'decentering' upon which Piaget puts so much emphasis as an indication of the level of cognitive growth achieved by the individual child. The *mentally retarded* children who were able to transform stimuli spent 50 per cent more time on the transformed item, a ratio of 1.5:1 (Note that this was not like the normals who were good transformers who gave equal time to both stimuli.) The mentally retarded children who were poor transformers were even more unusual with their line-of-sight behavior. They spent more than twice as long looking at the item on the display that they judged to be the greater of the two, a ratio of 2.4:1.

The training effects found by Wilton and Boersma are equally interesting. They have demonstrated that substantial effects are due to special experience, and that these improvements in ability to make the judgments were found in both normal and mentally retarded children. This diagnostic teaching, however, produced differential effects between the normals and the retarded when the line-of-sight records were analysed. The normals improved to a marked extent on the line-of-sight measures, whereas the mentally retarded children did not show such a definite improvement.

The present volume revives my interest in another unresolved controversy. To what extent are good transformers in the Piaget-type tasks found to be good at other transformation tasks, such as for instance reading? Farnham-Diggory and Bermon (1968) initiated this discussion when they noted that good transformers on the conservation-of-liquids task were twice as good as poor transformers when the children had to undertake the other task of transforming three pictorial elements into one combined action. Farnham-Diggory (1972) reminds us that this is a task which is closely related to early reading ability. But Hall, Salvi, Seggev, and Caldwell (1970) do not find these relationships. However, Professor Ruth Day of Yale University has several different unpublished studies which suggest that normal adult populations can be dichotomized into those who can undertake the transformation of ambiguous verbal materials presented either to the ears or the eyes, and those who cannot make such transformations. Perhaps we need to know more about the individual differences. Is it possible to use the differences in a more refined manner than simply transformers versus non-transformers? Are these marked differences responsible for the different results that the various investigators are finding on the relationship between the ability to transform in Piagetian tasks and achievement in other real-live tasks involving transformation of the presented stimuli?

Another source of ideas for future line-of-sight studies of anticipatory or achievement imagery is the Scottish work of Schaffer and Parry (1969) reported in Schaffer (1973). They found that they could demonstrate the presence of a stop-order on an action even at the age of 12 months. The point is that if we are to learn about the mechanisms whereby children switch to better strategies, then we may have to begin by learning more about how they use their internal imagery in relation to a new plan of action. The fact is that the beginning of wisdom may be in learning when not to act on a novel input. These authors compared how the 6 months old and 12 months old child reacts to a novel item. The visual orienting responses were found to be marked at both ages. But they also compared the tendency for the children to reach out immediately to the novel item. The young reached and touched the novel item without any delay. The year old children had learned to block that kind of impulsive reaction and checked their hand movements from reaching out at all. It took many trials for the older children to release this plan of action. Many linguistic responses much later in life involve the suppression of the immediate plan of action in favor of a more complex response which reacts to the combination of a number of elements rather than to each of the elements in turn.

The role of perceptual imagery in learning disabilities

Another question which cannot be solved without more basic investigations aimed at understanding the relation between the pictorial and language processing systems is that involving the nature of the breakdown which occurs when children cannot process verbal input in the form of spoken speech. These childhood aphasia cases give some insights into the role of a kind of imagery which does not seem to be anticipatory and therefore could perhaps be termed perceptual imagery. Again the evidence is of a preliminary nature, but it is mentioned here because these data were gathered by line-of-sight methods and emphasize that even the storage type of image can be impaired if the impairment is severe enough. The first point is that children who are severely affected with speech comprehension disorders have been shown to look for much longer periods at novel items appearing in the display. They continue to stare at this novel patch of color long after normal children have glanced at it for a few seconds and then moved their gaze to something else in the display. (Mackworth, Grandstaff, and Pribram, 1973). The thought is that possibly this phenomenon arises because such aphasic children may have trouble in forming the internal mental model of this external novelty and therefore they have to keep looking to keep on being informed. They are more stimulus-bound. Other studies have shown that even mildly impaired aphasic children take more than twice as long to decide that the correct visual symbol they are now looking at does indeed match the sample visual form, one second for aphasics and only half a second for normals (Grandstaff, Mackworth, de la Pena, and Pribram, 1974).

My point is the same as that mentioned earlier: if we assume that anticipatory images depend to some extent on the perceptual or storage imagery system working well, then it is necessary to examine the effectiveness of the perceptual imagery arrangements by, for instance, a match to sample task involving line-of-sight recording before concluding that it is a matter of the anticipatory imagery as such. This seems particularly important to add to studies involving mentally retarded persons because Spitz and Thor (1968) have already shown that letter processing is definitely slower than in normals of the same age. This was done with individual upper-case letters followed by a masking flash presented at various time intervals after the letter.

CONCLUSION

The Rotterdam University Press is to be congratulated in having such a handsome addition to their growing series of volumes on the problems related to learning disability.

H. Mackworth

REFERENCES

Bower, G.H., Mental imagery and associative learning; in Lee W. Gregg (Ed.), *Cognition in Learning and Memory*, New York, John Wiley and Sons, 1972, pp. 51–88.
Bruner, J.S., The course of cognitive growth, *American Psychologist*, 1964, *19*, 1–15.
Bryant, Discussion at Symposium on eye movements in child development, XXth International Congress of Psychology. Tokyo, 1972.

Cooper, R.M., The control of eye fixations by the meaning of spoken language, *Cognitive Psychology*, 1974, (in press).

Estes, W.K., *Learning Theory and Mental Development*, New York, Academic Press, 1970.

Farnham-Diggory, S., *Cognitive Processes in Education*, New York, Harper, 1972.
Farnham-Diggory, S. and M. Bermon, Verbal compensation, cognitive synthesis, and conservation, *Merrill-Palmer Quarterly*, 1968, *14*, 215–228.

Grandstaff, N.W., N.H. Mackworth, A. de la Pena and K.H. Pribram, *Visual matching by normal and speech disordered children*, 1974, (in preparation).

Hall, V.C., R. Salvi, L. Seggev, and E. Caldwell, Cognitive synthesis conservation, and task analysis, *Developmental Psychology*, 1970, *2*, 423–428.

Javal, E., Essai sur la physiologie de la lecture, *Annales d'oculistique*, 1878, *79*, 97. (ss Lévy-Schoen).

11

Lévy-Schoen, A. *L'Étude des Movements Oculaires*, Paris, Dunod, 1969.

Liberman, A.M., F.S. Cooper, D.P. Shankweiler, and M. Studdert-Kennedy, Perception of the speech code, *Psychological Review*, 1967, *74*, 341–461.

Mackworth, N.H., N.W. Grandstaff, and K.H. Pribram, Orientation to pictorial novelty by speech-disordered children, *Neuropsychologia*, 1973, (in press).

Myklebust, H., Indentification and diagnosis of children with learning disabilities; in S. Walzer & P. Wolff (Eds.), *Seminars in Psychiatry: Minimal Cerebral Dysfunction in Children*, New York, Grune and Stratton, 1973.

Paivio, A., *Imagery and Verbal Processes*, New York, Holt, Rinehart and Winston, 1971.

Osaka, R., An analysis of child development by eye-movement testing; in: *Abstract Guide of XXth International Congress of Psychology*, Tokyo, 1972.

Piaget, J., Piaget's Theory, in: P.H. Mussen (Ed.), *Carmichael's Manual of Child Psychology* (3rd ed.), New York, John Wiley and Sons, 1970., Vol. 1, pp. 703–732.

Piaget, J. and B. Inhelder, *Mental Imagery in the Child*, New York, Basic Books, 1971.

Pribram, K.H., *Languages of the Brain*, Englewood Cliffs, New Jersey: Prentice-Hall, 1971.

Rosenthal, W.S., J. Eisenson, and J.M. Luckau, A statistical test of the validity of diagnostic categories used in childhood language disorders: Implications for assessment procedures, in: D. Ingram (Ed.), *Papers and reports on child language development*, From Dr. E.V. Clark, Committee on Linguistics, Stanford University, Stanford, California, 94305, 1972.

Schaffer, H.R., The multivariate approach to early learning; in: R.A. Hinde & J. Stevenson-Hinde (Eds.), *Constraints on Learning*, New York, Academic Press. 1973. pp. 315–336.

Schaffer, H.R. and M.H. Parry, Perceptual-motor behaviour in infancy as a function of age and stimulus familiarity, *British Journal of Psychology*, 1969, *60*, 1–9.

Sheehan, P.W., *The Function and Nature of Imagery*, New York, Academic Press. 1973.

Spitz, H.H. and D.H. Thor. Visual backward masking in retardates and normals, *Perception and Psychophysics*, 1968, *4*, 245–246.

Vurpillot, E., The development of scanning strategies and their relation to visual differentiation, *Journal of Experimental Child Psychology*, 1968, *6*, 632–650.

Vurpillot, E., *Le Monde Visuel du Jeune Enfant*, Paris, Presses Universitaires de France, 1972.

Wedell, K., *Learning and Perceptuo-motor Disabilities in Children*, London, John Wiley and Sons, 1973.

Zeaman, D. and B.J. House, The role of attention in retardate discrimination learning, in: N.R. Ellis (Ed.), *Handbook of Mental Deficiency*, New York, McGraw-Hill, 1963, pp. 159–223.

1. Cognitive development and its assessment

INTRODUCTION

The possibility of accelerating the intellectual development of mentally retarded persons has been debated for many years. While a number of writers concerned with the education of the mentally retarded have expressed degrees of optimism regarding this issue (Itard, 1806; Seguin, 1866; Montessori, 1912; and notably Binet, 1909), a long-standing air of pessimism has also been apparent (Kirk, 1964). This is probably attributable to factors such as the widespread belief in the concept of a fixed intelligence (Hunt, 1961, 1969); the work of Goddard (1912) which seemed to imply that mental retardation reflected the influence of unalterable genetic factors; and Doll's (1941) widely accepted definition of mental retardation which included and emphasized a criterion of essential incurability. While this issue seems to be of basic methodological importance for psychology, it is by no means esoteric.

A recent study (Rosenthal & Jacobsen, 1968) has indicated that a teacher's expectations regarding normal children's potential intellectual ability can have a profound effect upon their subsequent intellectual development. Similar expectations on the part of parents, teachers, employers and institutional personnel are also likely to have a powerful influence upon the development of mentally retarded children. If this is so it is critical that these expectations should be optimistic, thus tending to facilitate rather than impede their cognitive development. Unless optimistic expectations have solid scientific support, however, they are unlikely to gain wider acceptance or to persist. Consequently, it seems important to find out whether or not the intellectual development of mentally retarded children, or aspects of it, can be accelerated by training or education.

Guskin and Spicker (1968) have reviewed a number of studies in which mentally retarded children have shown significant gains in I.Q. test scores following their participation in special education programs. A number of

13

measurement difficulties, however, (Lord, 1958; McNemar, 1940; Thorndike, 1966) make interpretation of differences in I.Q. test scores very difficult. And since conventional I.Q. tests are not based on systematic theories of intellectual development, it is difficult to relate I.Q. test score differences to intellectual development *per se.*

Piaget's (1947, 1970) theory of intellectual development attempts to account for changes in the nature of cognitive functioning during the development of the individual. The theory focuses on intraindividual differences which occur during development, rather than on interindividual differences which are present at a particular time (Elkind, 1969). Correlations between Piaget task performance and I.Q. test scores, however, are not high (Reese & Lipsitt, 1970), probably as these authors suggest, because Piaget tasks are limited to the assessment of cognitive functioning, whereas traditional I.Q. tests are designed to assess a number of other abilities that do not fall within the range of behaviors which Piaget (1947, 1970) classifies as intelligence (e.g., perceptual discrimination, verbal knowledge, etc.). While the relative usefulness of psychometric and Piagetian views of intelligence has yet to be determined, Piaget's view does appear to offer a promising alternative basis for research.

The acquisition of the notion of invariance or conservation, i.e., the realization that quantities remain invariant despite any spatial transformations they may undergo, has been extensively discussed by Piaget and his collaborators (Piaget, 1947; Piaget & Szeminska, 1941; Piaget & Inhelder, 1962, 1966). The acquisition of this notion is regarded as a significant indicator of intellectual development (Piaget, 1964a), and a reflection of the transition from preoperational to concrete operational thinking. Consequently, within this view of intellectual development, if a particular teaching strategy results in 'successful' acceleration of conservation the acceleration of this aspect of intellectual development may be presumed.

Piaget (1962) maintains that nonconservation is the surest evidence of preoperational thinking, and that the nonconserving child is reasoning from configurations estimating quantity from salient perceptual cues which are often unrelated to quantity. Furthermore, it is argued (Piaget, 1963a) that the nonconserver's reasoning lacks reversibility, thus enabling him to reason only about their transformations. Piaget maintains that the nonconserver's lack of reversibility arises because the child at this level centers on particular salient perceptual characteristics and is not able to *decenter* to other less salient, but more significant and relevant cues.

The transition from nonconservation to conservation according to Piaget (1947, 1959) follows four broad stages. Initially, the child attends to, and bases his reasoning on, configurational changes, i.e., changes in a

14

particular dimension or in the general shape of an array. Subsequently attention shifts to, and reasoning is based on, changes in the complementary dimension. Later attention and reasoning oscillate between dimensions, and awareness of the interdependence of dimensional changes begins to emerge. Finally, systematic scanning of both dimensions, together with an understanding of the principles of compensation, reversibility and identity, becomes apparent, and reasoning is now concerned with transformations.

Some variation is apparent with respect to the average ages at which particular conservation notions are acquired (conservation of number – 6-1/2 to 7 years; conservation of length – 7 to 8 years; conservation of continuous quantity (solids and liquids) – 7 to 8 years; conservation of volume – 11 to 12 years). Such notions are presumably mediated by similar cognitive structures. Piaget (1955) has invoked the concept of 'decalages horizontals' (horizontal differentials) to account for this relationship. As Wohlwill (1966) has observed, however, this concept is an ad hoc one and has probably not yet been adequately incorporated into Piaget's general theoretical position.

A large body of research has accumulated since Flavell's (1963) somewhat cautious review which seems to support the contention that the acquisition of conservation of number, length and continuous quantity (solid and liquid) can be accelerated through training (Beilin, 1971; Brainerd & Allen, 1971; Flavell & Hill, 1969). In addition, Gelman (1969) has reported successful acceleration of number and length conservation (over 95% success) and continuous quantity conservation (over 65% success) in five-year-old children as a function of number and length conservation training. Her findings were particularly interesting since the training effects were still present after a three week retention test interval.

A number of studies (e.g., Hood, 1962; Inhelder, 1963; Woodward, 1963) have indicated that mentally retarded children, in comparison with normals, progress through Piagetian developmental stages in the same sequence, but at a much slower rate and their upper level of operational development is less advanced. Within Piaget's (1947, 1970) theoretical scheme, the decentering of attention is a critical derivative of cognitive development. Thus, it seems highly probable that the relatively slow cognitive development of mentally retarded persons will be associated with attentional decentration difficulties (Wohlwill, 1966).

The possibility that there is a link between mental retardation and attentional problems has been recognized for many years (Crosby & Blatt, 1968), and has been underlined more recently by the work of Zeaman and House (1963), Luria (1963), and O'Connor and Hermelin

(1963). The question which arises is whether training aimed at influencing attentional processes might help overcome the developmental lag shown by mentally retarded children (Wohlwill, 1966). In this regard, Gelman (1969) has contended that nonconservers may fail to conserve because they do not attend to relevant cues, and that training can shape appropriate attentional behavior. If indeed a training procedure can shape attentional behavior which is necessary for conservation acquisition, it should thus be particularly appropriate for mentally retarded children.

Very few examinations have been made of conservation acceleration in mentally retarded children. In the first reported study, Brison and Bereiter (1967) attempted to accelerate solid and liquid quantity conservation, but it is difficult to interpret their findings. Although Piaget's criteria were used in defining pretraining nonconservation status, they were not used to define posttraining conservation acquisition. Posttraining conservation status was defined in terms of frequency of conservation judgements ('same' – following transformation) on conservation posttest tasks, and subsequent analyses of training errors and conservation explanations involved comparisons between conserving and nonconserving subjects defined in this way. No differences were observed between normals, gifted, and mildly retarded children in terms of conservation responses, or between normal, gifted or retarded 'conservers' in terms of explanations, either on posttests or transfer (within the same dimension) tasks. It is possible, however, and indeed likely that substantial intergroup posttraining differences may have existed. Some empirical support for this contention was provided by the authors, in that the retarded children did show a weak but significant trend in the direction of more rapid extinction of conservation responses following the presentation of evidence which apparently conflicted with the invariance (conservation) principle. Quite clearly, further investigation of this issue is required.

Subsequently, four additional acceleration studies have appeared. Schmalohr and Winkelmann (1969) reported successful though somewhat specific training effects in terms of quantity and substance conservation in normal and backward children. Lister (1969, 1970, 1972) used Piaget's criteria for defining pre and posttraining conservation status with educationally subnormal (midly retarded) children and reported successful acceleration of: weight conservation (1969); volume, area, substance, number, length, weight, and distance conservation (1970). On the basis of the above studies it would thus appear that the acquisition of conservation can be accelerated to a degree in mentally retarded children. Conservation acceleration studies, however, whether in normal or mentally retarded

16

children, entail methodological problems which permit differential interpretation of the results.

STRUCTURAL CHANGES AND THE PROBLEM OF THEIR ASSESSMENT

Although a number of writers have reported apparently successful acceleration of conservation, Piaget and his followers have argued that such results may be misleading, claiming that what has eventuated in many cases is pseudo-conservation (Inhelder, Bovet, Sinclair, & Smock, 1966; Piaget, 1967). Piaget has drawn a careful distinction between pseudo and true conservation. A child may be able to answer conservation questions correctly and still not be a 'true' conserver in Piaget's sense of the term (Piaget, 1964b). From Piaget's point of view, it is essential to establish that a child also has the necessary logical structures such as reversibility, compensation, etc., and can use these to deduce conservation as a necessary consequence of spatial transformations, before he can be described as a true conserver.

Piaget (1964a) has enumerated several criteria which may be used to evaluate training procedures and assess cognitive structural change. These are: *durability* or retention – the relative permanence of any changes which occur; *generalizability* or transfer – the extent to which training generalizes to new situations; and specification of the nature of cognitive structural changes which have occurred as a result of training. While the first two of these criteria seem to have been incorporated into most of the training studies reported to date, the third criterion raises several long-standing methodological difficulties. Verbal responses (changes in word meanings, language patterns, etc.) have been the traditional source of data on changes of this nature. The relationship between language and cognitive functioning, however, has proven extremely difficult to unravel (Berlyne, 1965; Furth, 1966; Piaget, 1954; Vygotsky, 1956). At the same time, verbal behavior seems to be highly responsive to experimenter cuing (Kingsley & Hall, 1968; Rosenthal, 1966), and some recent Russian research suggests that language and thinking are differentially related in mentally retarded and normal children (Shif, 1969).

Considerable disagreement has arisen regarding the effectiveness of various training procedures as evidenced by cognitive structural changes (Braine, 1959, Bruner, 1966; Piaget, 1967). Most of this dissent seems attributable to the ambiguity of verbal data. Piaget's (1964b, 1967) suggested extension of the conservation task does provide a check for pseudo-conservation. But as an index of cognitive structural change it does not seem entirely free of the above mentioned difficulties. Consequently, it would appear that some data in addition to changes in verbal behavior are required if less equivocal evidence of structural change is to be obtained.

Although cognitive structural changes presumably have a neurophysiological and chemical basis, analyses of this basis are clearly not possible given existing methods of study. Psychophysiological responses, however, appear to be one possible source of relevant nonverbal data. Moreover, such responses are probably less responsive than verbal data to experimenter cuing (O'Bryan & Boersma, 1971). Furthermore, since Piaget's usage of the term structure implies a continually modifying entity there seems good reason to suppose that an examination of ongoing psychophysiological activity should yield useful data on this question (Piaget, 1949, 1963b). If distinct differences in psychophysiological activity are apparent at various stages of conservation development, these measures should constitute useful evidence to supplement verbal data in the assessment of structural changes. Supplementary evidence of this nature should thus permit a more adequate evaluation of attempts to accelerate the acquisition of conservation.

Quite clearly, some aspects of psychophysiological functioning are more useful than others. Russian and Western researchers have indicated several variables which seem promising indicators of cognitive activity, viz., exploratory eye movements, galvanic skin response (GSR), vasomotor activity and heart rate (Berlyne, 1960, 1963, 1970; Creelman, 1966; Graham & Clifton, 1966; Gray, 1966; Lynn, 1966; Reese & Lipsitt, 1970). While Piaget's work is well known in the West and the USSR, and although psycho-physiological methods seem admirably suited for investigation into some of the questions which arise from Piaget's theoretical position (Jeffery 1968; Wright, 1963), to the authors' knowledge, no such research has yet been reported. In the present study, an attempt is made to develop psychophysiological indices of conservation acquisition which are used to supplement verbal data in examining conservation development and acceleration in normal and mentally retarded children.

According to Piaget's theoretical scheme a decrease in perceptual and cognitive centration is a critical derivative of the transition from preoperational to operational thinking. Consequently, there should be substantial differences in the cognitive functioning of conserving and nonconserving children and differential perceptual activity. This possibility was confirmed in a recent study in which corneally reflected eye movements were used as indices of perceptual activity, and a variety of distinct differences between conservers and nonconservers in terms of

18

eye-movement patterns were obtained (O'Bryan & Boersma, 1971). It was predicted that similar differences would be obtained in the present study between normal or retarded conservers and nonconservers, and if training was effective, between trained and untrained nonconservers.

Complementing the O'Bryan and Boersma study, the current investigation focused on two specific types of perceptual (eye-movement) activity. *General perceptual activity* was used to describe amount of overall visual exploratory activity. Piaget (1956) maintains that such activity tends to increase with age. It was predicted that normal and retarded conservers, and trained nonconservers (nonconservers who were to be trained), would show greater general perceptual activity during conservation task solution than nonconservers. Between group analyses were carried out on the general perceptual activity variables. *Centrative perceptual activity*, on the other hand, described the tendency to visually focus on specific elements. Piaget (1947) discusses a trend whereby perceptual and cognitive activity becomes decentered (attention becomes evenly displaced about the stimulus elements) with the onset of operational thinking, i.e., is no longer centered on particular states or dimensions of stimuli. It was predicted that normal and retarded conservers, and trained nonconservers, would show minimum centrative perceptual activity during conservation task solution, whereas maximum centrative perceptual activity would be associated with nonconservers. Within group analyses were undertaken on the centrative perceptual activity variables.

Charlesworth (1962, 1964, 1966) has obtained considerable support for his contention that children who understand a rule or principle will show surprise reactions when confronted with its apparent violation, whereas children who do not understand the rule or principle will not. Such findings may lead to the formulation of nonverbal estimates of cognitive structural development (Charlesworth, 1969), and thus may have considerable significance for developmental psychology. Presumably, surprise reactions would occur when prior expectancies regarding the outcome of the rule or principle in question are violated. Conversely, it seems probable that the occurrence of a surprise reaction following a violation of conservation is an indication that the cognitive structural changes which Piaget (1947) claims accompany conservation acquisition have taken place.

Apparent violations of conservation, and surprise reactions to them, have been used to assess conservation status by several other investigators (Achenbach, 1969; Mermelstein & Myer, 1969; Mermelstein & Shulman, 1967; Smedslund, 1961), although the results are difficult to interpret because of several methodological problems (Miller, 1971). A further problem with these studies stems from their use of predominantly verbal

19

surprise indices. For reasons outlined above, it is likely that nonverbal measures when used in conjunction with verbal measures would provide less ambiguous evidence of surprise. In this connection Lewis and Goldberg (1969) have shown that several psychophysiological components of the orientation reaction are elicited by young children following the violation of an expectancy. It seems likely that the occurrence of an orientation reaction following the violation of an expectancy reflects the significance of the violated relationship (level of cognitive structural development) for the children showing the orientation reaction (Lewis & Harwitz, 1969).

Achenbach's (1970) study with mentally retarded children indicated a close correspondence between verbal and GSR measures of surprise, following conservation violations. In view of the difficulty of distinguishing between orientation reactions and other psychophysiological reactions however (Lynn, 1966), it seems clear that multiple rather than single psychophysiological indices are to be preferred. The borderline between orientation and surprise reactions is extremely hazy (Charlesworth, 1969) but it seems clear from available research findings (Berlyne, 1960; Graham & Clifton, 1966; Gray, 1966; Lynn, 1966; Maltzman, 1967; Razran, 1961; Reese & Lipsitt, 1970; Sokolov, 1958, 1963), that the co-occurrence of a GSR, vasomotor activity, and cardiac deceleration, should follow the violation of expectancies during conservation tasks. In the present study, *surprise reactions* were thus defined as the simultaneous occurrence of a GSR conductance increase, a cephalic blood volume increase and a decrease in heart rate. It was surmised that conservers would expect that quantities do not change following spatial transformations, whereas nonconservers would expect that they do. Consequently, it was predicted that surprise reactions would be elicited by conservers, but not by nonconservers, in response to apparent violations of conservation.

In summary, the following considerations seem pertinent to the present investigation. Firstly, within Piaget's theory intellectual development is mirrored by a number of substantial changes in attentional behavior with a resulting trend towards decentration of thinking. Secondly, a number of researchers have documented the slower rate of cognitive development of mentally retarded persons with respect to Piagetian stages (e.g., Inhelder, 1963; Woodward, 1963). The association of attentional difficulties with mentally retarded persons has had a long history outside of the Piagetian theoretical framework (Crosby & Blatt, 1968), and since attentional behavioral change is a critical component of cognitive development within Piaget's scheme, it seems highly likely that attentional difficulties are strongly related to the slower rate of cognitive development in the mentally retarded.

Gelman (1969) has contended that nonconservers might become conservers if modifications in attentional behavior in the direction of maximum attention to task relevant cues could be induced. Moreover, she obtained some support for this contention. From Piaget's point of view, attention is mediated or controlled by existing cognitive structures. While the assumption that externally induced modifications in attentional behavior can lead to cognitive structural changes might seem at variance with an equilibration position, it is not necessarily so (Berlin, 1971), particularly with regard to the mentally retarded (Wohlwill, 1966). If training can induce appropriate attentional modifications with normal children it should also be effective with mentally retarded children. In addition, if modifications in attentional behavior can be accomplished which closely approximate those that occur in the normal developmental process, useful supplementary evidence bearing on cognitive structural change would seem to have been obtained. The use of perceptual activity and surprise reactions as well as verbal data in the present context should thus permit a more adequate examination of the possibility of conservation acceleration in mentally retarded and normal children.

SPECIFIC OBJECTIVES AND HYPOTHESES

In the present study, Piaget's definitional and training criteria were used in conjunction with perceptual activity variables and surprise reactions to examine the possibility of accelerating conservation acquisition in mildly retarded children. Since differential psychophysiological activity during cognitive processing in normal and retarded children is likely (Boersma, Wilton, Barham & Muir, 1970; Luria, 1963; Zeaman & House, 1963), it was first necessary to examine the above possibility as it relates to normal children. Furthermore, in order to evaluate obtained training effects, similar data from both normal and retarded natural (untrained) conservers and nonconservers is required. These comparisons were undertaken in a series of four studies.

Study 1 is an evaluation of the usefulness of general and centrative perceptual activity and surprise reactions, in conjunction with verbal data, for assessing the nature of cognitive structural differences between normal natural conservers and normal nonconservers.

The following hypotheses were tested in Study 1:

Hypotheses 1.1: Normal natural conservers, in comparison with non-conservers, will show greater general perceptual activity (more couplings, more runs, a shorter mean length of run, more fixations, and a shorter mean length of fixation) during the solution of conservation tasks.

Hypothesis 1.2: Normal natural conservers will show minimum centrative perceptual activity (no interelement differences in terms of frequency of runs, mean length of run, frequency of fixations, mean length of fixation, and percentage of examination time), during the solution of conservation tasks.

Hypothesis 1.3: Normal nonconservers will show maximum centrative perceptual activity (more runs, a greater mean length of run, more fixations, a greater mean length of fixation, and a greater percentage of examination time) on the element nominated as being greater in number, length or quantity, during the solution of conservation tasks.

Hypothesis 1.4: Normal natural conservers, in comparison with non-conservers, will show more surprise reactions and verbal awareness of legerdemain following apparent violations of conservation.

Hypothesis 1.5: Normal natural nonconservers will show a similar degree of centrative perceptual activity on conservation and conservation violation tasks, whereas natural conservers will show an increase in centrative perceptual activity on conservation violation tasks over that shown on conservation tasks.

Study 2 is an examination of the effectiveness of a conservation training procedure based on Gelman's (1969) technique, using Piaget's training criteria, and general and centrative perceptual activity and surprise reactions in conjunction with verbal data, for assessing the nature of cognitive structural differences between trained normal conservers (i.e., nonconservers who were to be trained) and normal nonconservers.

The following hypotheses were tested in Study 2:

Hypothesis 2.1: Trained normal conservers, in comparison with non-conservers, will show greater general perceptual activity during the solution of conservation tasks.

Hypothesis 2.2: Trained normal conservers will show minimum centrative perceptual activity during the solution of conservation tasks.

22

Hypothesis 2.3: Normal nonconservers will show maximum centrative perceptual activity during the solution of conservation tasks.

Hypothesis 2.4: Trained normal conservers, in comparison with non-conservers, will show more surprise reactions and verbal awareness of legerdemain following apparent violations of conservation.

Hypothesis 2.5: Normal nonconservers will show a similar degree of centrative perceptual activity on conservation and conservation violation tasks, whereas trained normal conservers will show an increase in centrative perceptual activity on conservation violation tasks over that shown on conservation tasks.

Study 3 is an evaluation of the usefulness of general and centrative perceptual activity and surprise reactions, in conjuction with verbal data, for assessing the nature of cognitive structural differences between mildly retarded natural conservers and mildly retarded nonconservers.

The following hypotheses were tested in Study 3:

Hypothesis 3.1: Midly retarded natural conservers, in comparison with nonconservers, will show greater general perceptual activity during the solution of conservation tasks.

Hypothesis 3.2: Mildly retarded natural conservers will show minimum centrative perceptual activity during the solution of conservation tasks.

Hypothesis 3.3: Mildly retarded nonconservers will show maximum centrative perceptual activity during the solution of conservation tasks.

Hypothesis 3.4: Mildly retarded natural conservers, in comparison with nonconservers, will show more surprise reactions and verbal awareness of legerdemain following apparent violations of conservation.

Hypothesis 3.5: Mildly retarded nonconservers will show a similar degree of centrative perceptual activity on conservation and conservation violation tasks, whereas mildly retarded natural conservers will show an increase in centrative perceptual activity on conservation violation tasks over that shown on conservation tasks.

Study 4 is an examination of the effectiveness of a conservation training procedure based on Gelman's (1969) technique, using Piaget's training criteria, and general and centrative perceptual activity and surprise reactions in conjunction with verbal data, for assessing the nature of cognitive structural differences between trained mildly retarded conservers (i.e., nonconservers who were to be trained) and mildly retarded nonconservers.

The following hypotheses were tested in Study 4:

Hypothesis 4.1: Trained mildly retarded conservers, in comparison with nonconservers, will show greater general perceptual activity during the solution of conservation tasks.

Hypothesis 4.2: Trained mildly retarded conservers will show minimum centrative perceptual activity during the solution of conservation tasks.

Hypothesis 4.3: Mildly retarded nonconservers will show maximum centrative perceptual activity during the solution of conservation tasks.

Hypothesis 4.4: Trained mildly retarded conservers, in comparison with nonconservers, will show more surprise reactions and verbal awareness of legerdemain following apparent violations of conservation.

Hypothesis 4.5: Mildly retarded nonconservers will show a similar degree of centrative perceptual activity on conservation and conservation violation tasks, whereas trained mildly retarded conservers will show an increase in centrative perceptual activity on conservation violation tasks over that shown on conservation tasks.

2. Outline of experimental method

GENERAL DESIGN

The children were pretested for number and length conservation at school and three normal groups (conservers, nonconservers to be trained, and nonconservers) and three retarded groups (as for normals) were selected. Each of the six respective subgroups contained 15 subjects, thus 45 normal and 45 retarded children were eventually used in the study. It should also be noted that the same groups of normal and retarded nonconservers were used, respectively, in Studies 1 and 2, and Studies 3 and 4. Figure 1 presents an outline of the experimental design.

The training groups received two training sessions on two consecutive mornings at school. In the afternoon following the second training session they were transported to the university where the experimental tasks were presented, and verbal and psychophysiological response data collected. Similar data were also collected at the university from the conserver and nonconserver groups. Three weeks after their laboratory visit the trained conserver and nonconserver groups were individually readministered the conservation posttests (number and length) and the conservation transfer tests (solid and liquid continuous quantity) at school.

An attempt was made to control for variations in intrasession history (Campbell, & Stanley, 1963) by dividing each of the six experimental groups into two subgroups each of which contained approximately half of the subjects. The resulting twelve subgroups were run in a counter-balanced order as follows:

a. Normal Conservers – Subgroup 1;
b. Normal Nonconservers – Subgroup 1;
c. Retarded Conservers – Subgroup 1;
d. Retarded Nonconservers – Subgroup 1;
e. Normal Trained Conservers – Subgroup 1;
f. Retarded Trained Conservers – Subgroup 1;
g. Retarded Trained Conservers – Subgroup 2;

h. Normal Trained Conservers – Subgroup 2;
i. Retarded Nonconservers – Subgroup 2;
j. Retarded Conservers – Subgroup 2;
k. Normal Nonconservers – Subgroup 2; and
l. Normal Conservers – Subgroup 2.

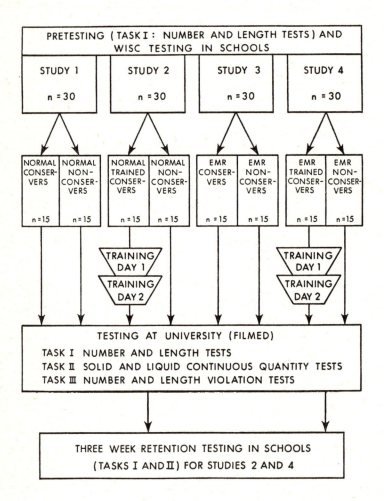

Figure 1. Outline of experimental procedure

26

Two populations from the local school system were involved in the present investigation, viz., mildly retarded and normal children. Mildly retarded subjects were defined as those children enrolled in elementary special classes scoring within the 50–85 range on the Wechsler Intelligence Scale for Children. These children were without known organic (neurological) defects and showed no evidence of sensory or emotional difficulties. Normal subjects were defined from a random sample of children attending regular first or second grade classes who also showed no evidence of sensory, emotional or organic difficulties.

Each child's school records were examined for medical data and children who deviated significantly from the standard 20/20 vision, or who showed auditory difficulties (2.72% of the normal subjects and 26.71% of the retarded subjects), were discarded from the respective sample populations. Since the corneal reflection eye-movement recording technique would not tolerate the reflective characteristics of glass, children requiring eye-glasses or contact-lenses were not included in the samples.

A total of 225 subjects (153 normals and 72 retardates) were individually administered the standard Piagetian pretests of number and length conservation at school. Subjects were required to give logical conservation responses on both tasks to be classified as conservers and conversely, nonconservation responses on both tasks to be classified as nonconservers. A subject who showed conservation behavior on one but not both tasks was classified as a transitional conserver and not used in the study. On this basis 73 normals were classified as conservers, 55 as nonconservers, and 25 transitional conservers. Of the retardates, there were 26 conservers, 43 nonconservers, and 3 transitional conservers. From the conserver pools, 15 normals and 15 retardates were selected at random. Similarly, 30 normals and 30 retardates were chosen from the nonconserver pools. The nonconservers were randomly assigned to training and control groups. An attempt was made to match sex ratios of all six groups as closely as possible. The mean age of the 45 normals (22 boys and 23 girls) in months was 82.82 with a range of 72–100 months, whereas for the 45 retardates (30 boys and 15 girls) it was, respectively, 119.86 and 87–145 months.

All subjects used in Studies 1, 2, 3 and 4 were administered the Wechsler Intelligence Scale for Children. The mean full scale I.Q. for the normal subjects was 109.60 (range 91–133) and for the retarded subjects 72.16 (range 55–82). An evaluation (Blishen, 1958) of socioeconomic status on the subjects used in the study indicated a predictably higher mean rank order rating for normals (mean = 3.84) than for retardates (mean = 5.39). All children lived in suburban areas of the city of Edmonton. The study was undertaken during January – April 1970.

APPARATUS

Eye movements were recorded by means of a Polymetric Model V-1164 eye-movement recorder. The recorder incorporates the use of corneal reflections superimposed upon a photograph of the stimulus material (Mackworth, 1967). The resultant corneally-reflected eye movements were filmed by a Pathé 'Professional' 16 mm. reflex movie camera at a constant exposure rate of 10 frames per second (see Figure 2).

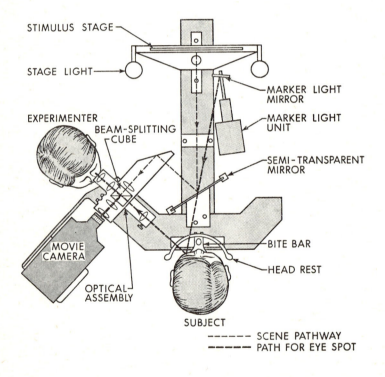

Figure 2. Schematic view of eye movement camera

A Grass Model 5 Polygraph, integrating a Model 5E DC driver-amplifier and Models 5P1 and 5P3 lowlevel DC preamplifiers, was used to obtain both GSR and plethysmographic recordings. For GSR measurement, zinc electrodes of 0.34″ in diameter were attached, using a zinc-sulphate paste, one to the central whorl on the distal-phalanx of the subject's thumb on the non-dominant hand, and the other to a lightly sanded area of skin on the volar surface of the subject's forearm (nondominant side), approximately 2″ from the wrist (Lykken, 1959). Plethysmographic recordings were obtained by a Grass Model RPT-1 (light reflected) photoelectric transducer, of the type described by Weinman (1967), which was attached to the subject's forehead approximately 2″ above the nose.

A 16 mm. L-W Photo-Optical Data Analyser Model 224-A was used for presenting the stimulus material. This projector permitted presentation of stop-action stimulus material, together with appropriate control frames, without interruption of the testing sequence. Task instructions were tape recorded and presented at a constant volume through head phones attached to a Sony four track tape recorder.

STIMULUS MATERIALS

Two rows of six 1-$\frac{1}{2}$″ diameter (i.e., 6 red and 6 blue) plastic poker chips were used for the number conservation pretest, while two 9″ × $\frac{3}{4}$″ strips of black cardboard were used for the length conservation pretest. Spatial transformations of these materials and those used in Tasks I and II were undertaken in the manner described by Piaget (1947).

Laboratory testing involved the movie presentation of conservation tasks. A previous study (O'Bryan & Boersma, 1972) has indicated that essential equivalent results can be expected from movie and traditional presentations of conservation tasks. The stimulus movie had three parts. First, the standard number and length conservation problems on which training had been given were shown (Task I); then followed two transfer problems, continuous quantity solid and liquid (Task II). Finally, a series of number and length conservation problems which appeared to violate the principle of conservation, together with appropriate control problems, were presented (Task III).

Task I problems (number conservation and length conservation) were identical to the pretest problems, except for their presentation via movie. The solid continuous quantity problem (Task IIa) involved the presentation of two balls of plasticine of 2″ diameter, one of which was rolled to form a sausage. In the liquid continuous quantity problem (Task IIb), two

29

8 oz. clear glass beakers each half filled with water were presented and the water in one of the beakers was poured into a higher and narrower 6 oz. clear glass beaker.

The final section of the film (Task III) consisted of a series of situations in which the principle of conservation, as it related to number (chips) and length (black cardboard strips) problems, was violated. In number conservation problems the number of chips increased in one of the rows when it was spread out, whereas in the length problems one of the cardboard strips lengthened as it was moved.

The assumption was made that conserving subjects would have strong expectations of conservation prior to a transformational sequence. However, the possibility existed that because of these strong expectations, a number of subjects might fail to perceive the conservation violations on their initial occurrence. Consequently, repeated presentation of these problems seemed necessary. In an attempt to avoid the occurrence of a set on the part of subjects towards an expectation of change in the quantity of the transformed stimulus, several control problems in which the quantity did not change (i.e., no deception was attempted) were included.

It seemed necessary to control for several factors in the Task III presentation order: viz., it needed to begin with violation instances of both number and length conservation; a violation instance needed to occur at the end of the series (a control problem would have served no purpose in this position); and the sequential occurrence of a long series of length or number problems was to be avoided. The following presentation order was designed with these factors in mind:

a. Number conservation violation (two rows of 6, changed to a row of 6 and a row of 8);
b. Length conservation violation (two 9″ strips of card were presented and one of these became 12″ long when it was moved);
c. Control problem (length);
d. Number conservation violation;
e. Control problem (number);
f. Control problem (length);
g. Length conservation violation;
h. Control problem (number);
i. Length conservation violation; and
j. Number conservation violation.

The three-week retention tests involved nonmovie presentation of Tasks I and II.

The training procedure was, except for one modification (stimuli were presented pictorially rather than in concrete form), essentially identical to that developed and described in detail by Gelman (1969). The children were presented individually a series of 32 six-trial oddity learning problems in which number and length were relevant cues on alternate problems. Training was undertaken on two consecutive days with 16 problems presented in each session. The problems were presented pictorially on 10" × 8" sheets of white cardboard.

For each trial three stimuli were presented, and in each case two stimuli were equivalent (either in length or number, depending on the problem) and the other differed on the same dimension (either shorter or longer, more or less). The subject was required to indicate either two stimuli which were the same, or two which were different. Between, but not within, problem variations included color (red, yellow, green, or blue), shape (round or square), size (small or large), and spatial position (horizontal, vertical, a combination of horizontal and vertical, or geometric patterns).

Gelman's procedure was used to vary systematically the salience of relevant and irrelevant cues within each problem. All cues were relevant and redundant on Trial 1 while alignment and geometric cues varied independently of number and/or length cues on Trials 2–5. On Trial 6 irrelevant cues were held constant and if a response was to be correct it would need to have been made on the basis of relevant quantitative relationships, i.e., number (number problems) or length (length problems) between the stimuli. A child was considered to have learned the number and length problems if he made no more than one error for each of the last two problems. All normal and retarded children reached this criterion for both types of problems.

DEFINITIONS AND DEPENDENT VARIABLES

Periods

Stimulus transformation period: the period of time varying from 7.0 to 13.5 seconds during which the filmed transformation was presented.

Decision period: the period of time from which the outcome of the stimulus transformation becomes apparent until the subject responds to a particular conservation or conservation violation problem by closing his eyes.

Decision latency: the amount of time in one-tenth second units that it takes subject to respond to the question.

Prefilm period: the five second period immediately preceding the movie presentation of each conservation or conservation violation problem.

Transformation outcome period: the period of time from the point at which the outcome of the stimulus transformation becomes visible until five seconds after the completion of the transformation. This period varied with tasks (6.5 to 9.0 seconds) but was approximately standard across subjects.

Eye movement terms

Fixation: one or more successive corneal reflections recorded at a rate of 10 frames per second within the same circular area subtended by 15 minutes of arc in the stimulus field. Specifically, the point at which the subject concentrates his gaze for a minimum period of one-tenth of a second while eye movements are being recorded.

Run: two or more consecutive fixations exclusively on either the transformed or nontransformed stimulus element.

Coupling: a shift in fixation from one stimulus element to the other, i.e., a probable comparison between the transformed and nontransformed elements.

Frequency of couplings: the total number of comparisons made between the elements.

Frequency of runs: the total number of runs made on the transformed element, nontransformed element, or summed over both elements.

Frequency of fixations: the total number of shifts in fixation (plus one) on the transformed element, nontransformed element, or summed over both elements.

Mean length of run: the ratio of the summated number of one-tenth second units in all runs to the summated number of runs made on the transformed element, nontransformed element, or summed over both elements.

Mean length of fixation: the ratio of the summated number of one-tenth second units to the summated total number of fixations on the transformed element, nontransformed element, or summed over both elements.

Examination time: the summated total number of one-tenth second units, on either the transformed or nontransformed elements, or summed over both elements.

Psychophysiological terms

GSR conductance increase: a noticeable upward deflection in the GSR record during the transformation outcome period, i.e. a decrease in skin resistance during this period.

Blood volume increase: an increase in mean cephalic blood volume flow during the transformation outcome period over that observed in the prefilm period.

Heart rate increase: an increase in beats per minute during the transformation outcome period over that observed in the prefilm period.

Surprise reaction: the simultaneous occurrence during the transformation outcome period of a GSR conductance level increase, a mean cephalic blood volume increase, and a beats per minute heart rate decrease.

TESTING PROCEDURE

After conservation pretesting the children were transported (four per day) to the university for the eye-movement recording session. Here they were fitted with a bite-bar to minimize head movements during eye-movement recording and seated comfortably at the apparatus. The GSR electrodes and photo-electric transducer were also attached at this time. The eye-movement recorder was then positioned and calibrated, and Tasks I, II, and III administered.

Tasks I, II, and III were presented on 16 mm. black and white movie film which was rear-projected on to a 7.8" × 7.8" stimulus viewing screen. The screen was positioned on a horizontal plane approximately 24" in front of the subject's eyes. In an attempt to standardize presentation techniques, facilitate filming eye movements and collection of GSR and plethysmographic data, the movie presentations were synchronized with taped verbal instructions. In addition, before any data was collected, a series of 35 mm. slides of 'Stanford-Binet Picture Absurdity Tasks' was presented to the subjects who were trained to close their eyes when they had solved each problem.

Because pilot investigations had indicated consistently strong psychophysiological reactions to taped verbal instructions in both normal and retarded subjects, and because the present study was additionally concerned with the presence or absence of such reactions as a function of the various stimulus transformations, a minor modification in the questioning procedure of O'Bryan and Boersma (1971) was necessary. Whereas in their study the conservation question was asked immediately following the

33

stimulus transformation, in the present study subjects were questioned prior to stimulus transformation. It should be noted that the experimental task was not one of prediction. Subjects were asked for their responses to a conservation question only after the particular transformation had been completed and the subjects had signalled their decision with eye-closure. Thirty subjects were selected at random from the experimental population, and a check was made for retention across the question – decision interval. No forgetting of the question was apparent in any of the treatment groups.

Within Task I, the number conservation problem was followed by the length problem. Conservation questions, as previously mentioned, were asked prior to the stimulus transformation period, with subjects being instructed to close their eyes when they had reached a post-transformation decision as to whether the two elements were the same or different. Eye-movements were recorded from the point at which the stimulus transformation outcome became apparent until children closed their eyes, i.e. during the decision period. Verbal responses were then tape-recorded. The same eye-movement recording procedure was followed during the presentation of Task II, with the solid and liquid continuous quantity problems being presented in that order, and in Task III. Psychophysiological (surprise reaction) data were collected for Task III during the transformation outcome period.

SCORING PROCEDURE

The first three seconds (30 frames) of eye-movement data were scored for each subject in terms of fixations on the transformed and nontransformed elements. A number of frames, however, (less than 3%), were present in which the corneal reflection was indefinable, blurred, or not apparent (e.g., as a result of a blink, a very rapid eye movement, or a looking away from the stimulus field). The scoring of these frames was estimated as follows:

All fixation points in the first half of a sequence of frames (X) which was to be interpolated were estimated as being in the same area as the fixation point immediately preceding X. All fixation points in the latter half of X were estimated as being in the same area as the fixation point immediately following X. Where X was an odd number of frames, the extra frame was added to the second half of X. It was decided that any subject who showed more than 10% of interpolated data on any task item would be eliminated from the study. No subjects were eliminated on this basis. A random sample of 20 eye-movement and psychophysiological records were analyzed independently by two judges. There was over 95% agreement in the eye-movement data.

Psychophysiological (surprise reaction) data were scored relative to change during the transformation outcome period, irrespective of decision latency. In that it took 4 seconds to complete the transformation for number problems once the outcome was apparent, and only 1.5 seconds for length problems, the transformation outcome periods, respectively, for number and length items were 9.0 and 6.5 seconds. The five second interval, added at the point of transformation completion, was included to allow time for the surprise reaction to occur. This gave a slightly longer time base to number problems, but an approximately standard time interval for problems across subjects.* GSR, heart rate, and blood volume were scored as positive (a change in predicted direction) only when two judges agreed on the classification. More than 85% of the items analyzed were the first presented ones. Furthermore, there was no difference in percentage of first presented items scored as a function of type of problem or group.

CORRELATIONS BETWEEN EYE MOVEMENT VARIABLES

Pearson product-moment correlation coefficients were determined among the five general perceptual activity variables (frequency of couplings, frequency of runs, mean length of run, frequency of fixations, and mean length of fixation) and the five centrative perceptual activity variables (i.e., ratio differences between the transformed and nontransformed elements for frequency of runs, mean length of run, frequency of fixations, mean length of fixation and amount of examination time), and between general perceptual activity and centrative perceptual activity variables. General perceptual activity measures correlated positively (or in the expected direction) with each other as did centrative perceptual activity measures, with 50% of the correlations in each classification being 0.50 or higher. And all intercorrelations between general perceptual activity and centrative perceptual activity measures were negative, al-

* It appears unlikely that eye closure could account for surprise reaction differences in favor of conservers and trained conservers discussed later since these groups had on the average longer decision latencies than the nonconservers. Where decision latencies were shorter than the transformation outcome period (approximately 31% of the normal and 44% of the retardate observations), data were scored in terms of the decision period.

35

though not strongly so. Thus, the above results support the general and centrative perceptual activity classifications used in the present series of studies.

STATISTICAL ANALYSES

A 2 × 2 factorial analysis of variance design with repeated measures on the second factor (Winer, 1962), was used for testing between group hypotheses. Groups (conserver or trained nonconserver vs nonconserver) was the nonrepeated factor, and Tasks (I and II for Hypotheses 1.1, 2.1, 3.1, and 4.1) the repeated measures. The z test for independent proportions (Ferguson, 1966) was used for testing Hypotheses 1.4., 2.4, 3.4, and 4.4.

Within group Hypotheses 1.2, 1.3, 1.5; 2.2, 2.3, 2.5; 3.2, 3.3, 3.5; and 4.2, 4.3, 4.5 were tested using the t test for correlated samples (Winer, 1962). In Studies 2 and 4 frequency of logical conservation responses on Tasks I and II, in both laboratory tests and three week retention tests, were compared using the z test for independent proportions.*

---

* All t and z tests of experimental hypotheses involved one-tailed comparisons.

3. Results and discussion

Results

Conservers tended to take longer than nonconservers to reach task decisions and the data were therefore analyzed over a constant time interval rather than in terms of decision latencies. Previous eye-movement research (Boersma, Muir, Wilton & Barham, 1969; O'Bryan & Boersma, 1971) suggested that the first three seconds of the decision period was a meaningful time base from which to analyze such data. The frequency of unscorable frames and percentage of missing data (from short decision latencies) were also minimal during this period. Consequently, it was decided to adopt this unit as the constant time interval for analyses of the eye-movement data.

Conservation tasks

Eye-movement data. A Tasks (I and II) by Groups (conservers and nonconservers) analysis of variance with repeated measures on Tasks was used for between group analyses of general perceptual activity. The following results were obtained. Conservers, in comparison with nonconservers, showed more couplings ($\bar{X}_{nc} = 3.42$, $\bar{X}_{nnc} = 1.79$; $F = 15.373$, $df = 1/28$, $p < .001$)*, more runs summed over both elements ($\bar{X}_{nc} = 2.14$, $\bar{X}_{nnc} = 1.69$; $F = 4.516$, $df = 1/28$, $p < .05$), and a shorter mean length of run in one tenth second units summed over both elements ($\bar{X}_{nc} = 12.83$, $\bar{X}_{nnc} = 18.33$; $F = 13.045$, $df = 1/28$, $p < .01$), more fixations over both elements ($\bar{X}_{nc} = 10.87$, $\bar{X}_{nnc} = 8.15$; $F = 12.329$, $df = 1/28$, $p < .01$), and a

---

* Lower case letters nc and nnc associated with mean values refer, respectively, to normal conservers and normal nonconservers.

shorter mean length of fixation in one tenth second units over both elements ($\bar{X}_{nc}$ = 3.11, $\bar{X}_{nnc}$ = 4.19; F = 10.491, df = 1/28, p < .01). No significant Task or interaction effects were obtained. Thus, Hypothesis 1.1 is supported and a clear differentiation between normal conservers and normal nonconservers in terms of general perceptual activity seems indicated.

Within group differences of task performance in relation to the transformed and nontransformed elements on Tasks I and II were analysed using correlated t tests. For each subject data was summed over problems (i.e., over problems Ia, Ib, IIa and IIb) and divided by four. These scores were then used as raw scores from which group means for the correlated t tests were calculated. Table 1 summarizes these results.*

Table 1. Summary of correlated t tests on Tasks I and II eye movement data for normal subjects

	Nonconservers			Trained Conservers			Conservers		
	GE$\bar{X}$[a]	LE$\bar{X}$[b]	t	TE$\bar{X}$[c]	NTE$\bar{X}$[d]	t	TE$\bar{X}$	NTE$\bar{X}$	t
Number of runs	1.50	1.07	2.34*	1.68	1.55	0.52	1.67	1.47	0.60
Mean length of run	20.64	12.77	1.97*	14.17	14.13	0.01	11.44	13.00	0.52
Number of fixations	7.60	4.82	2.59*	8.55	7.72	0.77	8.00	8.28	0.25
Mean length of fixation	5.76	4.37	1.85*	4.29	3.91	1.03	4.34	3.93	0.89
Amount of examination time	23.73	14.40	2.28*	19.28	17.60	0.49	17.05	16.48	0.15

[a]GE$\bar{X}$ Mean value on element chosen as greater
[b]LE$\bar{X}$ Mean value on element chosen as lesser
[c]TE$\bar{X}$ Mean value on transformed element
[d]NTE$\bar{X}$ Mean value on nontransformed element
* $p < .05$

The analyses revealed that nonconservers made significantly more runs on the greater element (t = 2.34), df = 14, p < .05), had a longer mean length of run in one tenth second units on the greater element (t = 1.97,

* In Tables 1 and 3 the terms GE (greater element) and LE (lesser element) are used to denote the elements erroneously perceived by the nonconservers as greater and lesser in quantity. Two normal and two mildly retarded nonconservers perceived the nontransformed element as greater, and for these four subjects GE dependent variable measures refer to nontransformed element data.

38

$df = 14, p < .05$), made significantly more fixations on the greater element ($t = 2.59, df = 14, p < .05$), had a longer mean length of fixation in one tenth second units on the greater element ($t = 1.85, df = 14, p < .05$) and spent a significantly larger amount of examination time (tenths of seconds) on the greater element ($t = 2.28, df = 14, p < .05$). Similar analyses for conservers, however, failed to yield significant differences.

These results provide support for Hypotheses 1.2 and 1.3, thus suggesting that conserving and nonconserving subjects showed clearly different patterns of centrative perceptual activity. Whereas nonconservers appeared to center their perceptual activity on the particular element perceived to be greater in number, length, or quantity, following transformation, conservers did not.

Violation Tasks. Analyses of these data are presented in two sections:
a. in terms of the variables which seem most crucial to this aspect of the study, namely, verbal reports and surprise reactions; and
b. in terms of within group analyses of eye-movement data, i.e., inter-element comparisons.

A comparison between the conserver and nonconserver groups on verbal responses to violation items revealed that all of the conservers attributed the apparent conservation violations to some legerdemain, whereas only 16% of the nonconservers responded in this way ($z = 6.56$, $p < .0001$). A substantially higher percentage of surprise reactions (the simultaneous occurrence during the transformation outcome period of a GSR conductance increase, a cephalic blood volume increase and a heart rate decrease) were also observed for conservers (53% vs. 17%; $z = 2.98$, $p < .005$). Thus Hypothesis 1.4 was strongly supported. Moreover, in view of the intergroup differences on verbal responses, it would appear that the occurrence of surprise reactions closely reflects the recognition of conservation violations.

A summary of within group analyses of eye movement data on Task III, is presented in Table 2. The results indicate with respect to the transformed and nontransformed elements that conservers made more runs on the transformed element ($t = 3.68, df = 14, p < .01$), had a significantly longer mean length of run in one tenth second units on the transformed element ($t = 2.93, df = 14, p < .01$), made more fixations on the transformed element ($t = 5.13, df = 14, p < .001$), had a longer mean length of fixation in one tenth second units on the transformed element ($t = 1.96$, $df = 14, p < .05$), and spent a greater amount of examination time (tenths of seconds) on the transformed element ($t = 3.70, df = 14$, $p < .01$). Nonconservers showed a significantly longer mean length of run in one tenth second units on the transformed element ($t = 1.95$, $df = 14$, $p < .05$), and more fixations on the transformed element ($t = 1.94$, $df = 14$, $p < .05$), but none of the other differences were significant.

Table 2. Summary of correlated t tests on Task III eye movement data for normal subjects

	Nonconservers			Trained Conservers			Conservers		
	TE$\overline{X}$[a]	NTE$\overline{X}$[b]	t	TE$\overline{X}$	NTE$\overline{X}$	t	TE$\overline{X}$	NTE$\overline{X}$	t
Number of runs	1.43	1.10	1.11	1.53	1.23	1.26	1.97	1.17	3.68**
Mean length of run	22.90	11.26	1.95*	21.12	12.65	1.63	24.91	9.01	2.93**
Number of fixations	8.60	5.23	1.94*	9.07	6.07	1.81*	12.77	5.67	5.13***
Mean length of fixation	4.22	2.83	1.70	4.53	3.53	1.52	3.85	2.40	1.96*
Amount of examination time	26.00	14.80	1.73	23.73	14.67	1.65	30.37	11.23	3.70**

[a]TE$\overline{X}$ Mean value on transformed element
[b]NTE$\overline{X}$ Mean value on nontransformed element
* $p < .05$
** $p < .01$
*** $p < .001$

Inspection of Table 1 in conjunction with Table 2 reveals that nonconservers tend to center on the transformed element in both cases with the strongest effect being associated with Table 1. More interesting, however, is the marked contrast evident in the case of conservers. Here, for Task III, all dependent variables showed significant interelement differences in favor of the transformed element, whereas none were significant on Table 1. Support was thus obtained for Hypothesis 1.5 in that conservers showed an increase in centrative perceptual activity, whereas nonconservers did not.

In summary, the following results emerged from Study 1. Conservers in comparison with nonconservers showed predicted differences in general and centrative perceptual activity on conservation tasks. Predicted intergroup differences in verbal responses and surprise reactions to conservation violations were also obtained, and in conservers these reactions were accompanied by predicted changes in centrative perceptual activity.

Discussion

The results of between and within group analyses of Task I and II eye-movement data provided strong support for the experimental hypotheses. These findings appear to indicate that in terms of corneally reflected eye movements the general perceptual behavior of conservers is considerably more active than that of nonconservers, and that the lesser perceptual activity of nonconserving subjects is accompanied by a tendency on their part to *center* or fixate significantly longer and more often on the element judged to be greater following transformation. These results seem consistent with Piaget's (1947, 1970) distinctions between the perceptual/attentional concomitants of preoperational and operational thinking, and replicate the findings of O'Bryan and Boersma (1971).

The conservation violation tasks also differentiated the groups in the predicted direction. The marked differences between the groups in terms of their verbal responses to the apparent violations of conservation suggest that the expectancies of the conservers and nonconservers with respect to the possible transformation outcome were very different prior to the completion of the transformation. All of the conservers reported that something wrong had occurred and they attributed the violation to legerdemain. On the other hand, almost all of the nonconservers gave the usual nonconservation response and rationale.

The differences between the groups in terms of surprise reactions indicate that during the transformation outcome period on conservation violation tasks psychophysiological activity differentiated conserving and nonconserving subjects. With respect to eye movements the within group analyses of Task III data revealed a number of marked changes in the conservers' centrative perceptual activity, whereas little or no change was apparent in nonconservers. As predicted, the changes in conservers' centrative perceptual activity involved substantial increases in interelement differences for the five ratios. Moreover, number of runs, mean length of run, number of fixations, and percentage of time spent looking at the transformed element, i.e., the element which was manipulated to appear greater, all increased.

Although the centrative perceptual activity of conservers on Task III appeared to be similar to that shown by nonconservers there were probably very different reasons for each group's performance. Nonconservers probably showed more perceptual activity on the transformed element because, as in conservation tasks, this element appeared to be greater (Piaget, 1961) following transformation. In the case of conservers, however, the increase in perceptual activity on the transformed element was probably a function of their recognition of conservation violation.

The obtained results provide considerable support for Charlesworth's (1969) and Lewis and Harwitz's (1969) contentions regarding the utility of surprise and orientation reactions as nonverbal indices of cognitive structural change. Piaget's (1947, 1962, 1970) position is also strongly supported in that there appear to be marked differences in the cognitive functioning of conserving and nonconserving subjects following apparent conservation violations. Presumably, surprise reactions are centrally mediated and it seems highly likely that the occurrence of such reactions following conservation violation closely reflects cognitive structural changes associated with conservation attainment. General and centrative perceptual activity and surprise reaction data thus seems to be useful supplementary indicators of cognitive structural development. Moreover, when accompanied by verbal data, they may lead to a more adequate evaluation of conservation acceleration attempts.

STUDY 2. PERCEPTUAL ACTIVITY AND SURPRISE REACTIONS IN TRAINED NORMAL CONSERVERS AND NORMAL NONCONSERVERS

Results

Conservation tasks: verbal data. Substantial intergroup differences were evident on immediate posttests. On Tasks I (direct transfer from training) and II (indirect transfer) trained normal conservers showed a significantly higher proportion of logical conservation responses than nonconservers (Task I: 80% vs. 00%, $z = 7.81$, $p < .0001$; Task II: 47% vs. 00%, $z = 4.87$, $p < .0001$). A similar pattern arose on three week retention tests. Here trained conservers also showed more logical conservation responses than nonconservers on Task I (77% vs. 3%, $z = 5.79$, $p < .0001$) and Task II (53% vs. 00%, $z = 4.61$, $p < .0001$). These results were supportive of Gelman's (1969) findings, and it would appear in terms of generalizability (indirect transfer) and permanence (three week retention) that the training procedure was successful. More detailed analyses of cognitive structural changes in terms of eye movement and surprise reaction data thus seemed meaningful and were undertaken.

Conservation tasks: eye-movement data. In general, trained normal conservers were slower to reach task decisions than were normal nonconservers, and as in Study 1, the analysis of eye movement data in terms of a constant time interval was indicated for both conservation and violation tasks. The first three seconds of the decision period was again adopted for this purpose.

A two-way (Groups by Tasks) analysis of variance with repeated measures on Tasks (I & II) was used for between group analyses of eye-movement data. The following results were obtained. In comparison with normal nonconservers, the trained normal conservers showed more couplings* ($\bar{X}_{nt} = 2.90$, $\bar{X}_{nnc} = 1.79$; $F = 9.493$, $df = 1/28$, $p < .01$), more runs summed over both elements ($\bar{X}_{nt} = 2.17$, $\bar{X}_{nnc} = 1.69$; $F = 6.316$, $df = 1/28$, $p < .05$), a shorter mean length of run in one tenth second units ($\bar{X}_{nt} = 13.10$, $\bar{X}_{nnc} = 18.33$; $F = 10.555$, $df = 1/28$, $p < .01$), more fixations over both elements ($\bar{X}_{nt} = 10.55$, $\bar{X}_{nnc} = 8.15$; $F = 7.404$, $df = 1/28$, $p < .05$) and a shorter mean length of fixation in one tenth second units over both elements ($\bar{X}_{nt} = 3.27$, $\bar{X}_{nnc} = 4.19$; $F = 6.462$, $df = 1/28$, $p < .05$). Both groups also showed more fixations on Task I ($\bar{X}_{I} = 9.98$, $\bar{X}_{II} = 8.72$, $F = 4.301$, $df - 1/28$, $p < .05$). No other Task or interaction effects were significant. Thus for all practical purposes trained conservers showed the same type of general perceptual activity as that of conservers in Study 1. Consequently, Hypothesis 2.1 is supported, and marked differences between trained conservers and nonconservers with respect to general perceptual activity are evident.

Correlated t tests were used for within group analyses of eye-movement data in relation to the transformed and nontransformed elements on Tasks I and II. For each subject data was summed over problems (i.e., problems Ia, Ib, IIa and IIb) and divided by four as in Study 1. These results are summarized in Table 1. Since the same nonconserver subjects were used for comparative purposes in Study 2 and in Study 1, nonconserver results are identical to those reported in Study 1. None of the interelement differences for trained conservers were significant. Thus distinct intergroup differences in centrative perceptual activity are evident and Hypotheses 2.2 and 2.3 are supported. The more interesting finding, however, is that centrative perceptual activity of trained and natural conservers is very similar, indicating that eye-movement patterns of trained conservers closely resemble those of natural conservers.

Violation tasks. Verbal responses to violation items clearly differentiated the groups. Significantly more trained conservers than nonconservers attributed the apparent conservation violations to legerdemain ($\bar{X}_{nt} = 73\%$, $\bar{X}_{nnc} = 16\%$; $z = 4.41$, $p < .0001$). It would appear therefore that

---

* Lower case letters nt and nnc are used to refer, respectively, to normal trained conservers and normal nonconservers.

trained conservers and nonconservers had differential expectations with respect to the transformation outcome. Trained conservers also showed significantly more surprise reactions than nonconservers (43% vs. 17%; $z = 2.25$, $p < .025$), thus supporting Hypothesis 2.4. A similar trend to that obtained in Study 1 seems evident. The occurrence of surprise reactions again appears to be related to conservation violation recognition.

Within group analyses of Task III eye-movement data in terms of the transformed and nontransformed elements are summarized in Table 2. Here trained conservers showed more fixations on the transformed element ($t = 1.81$, $df = 14$, $p < .05$), an effect which was not noticeable for Task I and II (see Table 1). Table 2 also shows two interelement differences for nonconservers, in contrast to the five significant differences which are apparent in Table 1. Inspection of nonconservers data in Table 2 shows, however, that although only two interelement differences are significant, the larger mean measures of centrative perceptual activity are in all cases associated with the transformed element. Thus, these results do in fact parallel those associated with the greater element in Table 1. Therefore Hypothesis 2.5 received some support. Trained conservers did show an increase in number of fixations on the transformed element (a slight change in centrative perceptual activity) whereas nonconservers tended to continue to focus on the transformed element, i.e., the element that originally appeared greater. The fact remains, however, that four out of five interelement comparisons for trained conservers on Task III were not significant and that their eye-movement behavior in terms of these analyses was different from that of natural conservers. Therefore these findings should be interpreted with caution.

A more detailed comparison of Task I and II results (Table 1) with Task III results (Table 2) for trained conservers revealed several interesting changes in perceptual activity in relation to the transformed and nontransformed elements. Specifically, on Task III all transformed element measures, except number of runs, increased. Also, overall number of runs were fewer on Task III, but the ratio between all transformed and nontransformed element measures increased. Thus it appears that trained conservers noticed the conservation violation and modified their perceptual behavior accordingly, whereupon their perceptual activity became somewhat similar to that shown by the nonconservers.

In summarizing the results of Study 2, the following points seem important. Trained conservers and nonconservers showed predicted differences in general and centrative perceptual activity on conservation tasks on Tasks I and II. On conservation violation tasks, predicted intergroup differences in verbal responses and surprise reactions were also

44

obtained, and in trained conservers on Task III these reactions were accompanied by some predicted changes in centrative perceptual activity.

Discussion

Strong support was obtained for the hypotheses relating to general and centrative perceptual activity on Tasks I and II in that distinct intergroup differences were apparent. Trained conservers showed more active general perceptual behavior than nonconservers, and while nonconservers showed a marked tendency to center more often and for longer periods on the element judged to be greater following the transformation, such a trend was not apparent with respect to either element in trained conservers. Therefore, in addition to verbal response data, analyses of general and centrative perceptual activity during Tasks I and II seemed to provide considerable support for the contention that the conservation acceleration procedure had been effective in inducing a degree of cognitive structural change in the trained conservers.

The intergroup differences in verbal and surprise reactions to apparent conservation violations also provided support for the effectiveness of the conservation acceleration procedure in terms of cognitive structural changes. Significantly more trained conservers than nonconservers recognized the apparent conservation violations, thus suggesting that prior to transformation completion the expectancies of the two groups with respect to the transformation outcome were very different. Furthermore, trained conservers showed significantly more surprise reactions than nonconservers. It seems very likely the above data reflects a higher percentage of perceived violations of pretransformation expectancies on the part of trained conservers.

Within group analyses of Task III eye-movement data in comparison with Task I and II data also provided some support for the contention that the conservation acceleration procedure was effective in terms of inducing cognitive structural change. These findings, however, were less supportive than previous ones and difficult to interpret.

With reference to Study 1 (Tasks I and II), general and centrative perceptual activity in natural and trained conservers appear essentially equivalent, and both contrast with that shown by nonconservers. In addition, verbal and surprise reaction frequencies in both studies were substantially greater than those shown by nonconservers. Natural and trained conservers also showed somewhat similar eye-movement patterns during Task III, although the similarities were not as pronounced as those observed on Tasks I and II.

45

Consequently, training appeared to be effective. Moreover, in terms of verbal, eye-movement and surprise reaction data it appeared that cognitive structural development of trained conservers closely paralleled that shown by natural conservers. It is difficult, however, to make comparisons between trained and natural conservers since the analyses of verbal data on conservation tasks indicates that training was not equally effective for all subjects. For example, some subjects showed conservation responses on Task I but not on Task II, or showed Task II conservation responses immediately following training but not after three weeks. Thus, in some cases training probably resulted in pseudoconservation behavior. Since the training group data included observations on these subjects and on those who gave nonconservation responses for both Tasks I and II immediately following training, training effects may actually have been suppressed. Therefore, it appeared interesting to compare eye-movement, surprise reaction and verbal response data to conservation violation tasks from the eight subjects for whom training was apparently successful with that from the seven subjects who either failed to conserve or appeared to show pseudoconservation acquisition.

Such a comparison, in general, suggested that general perceptual behavior was less active in unsuccessful subjects. For the unsuccessful group 58% of the relevant observations were below the training group means (or in the case of duration of runs and fixations, were above the training group means) used in the analyses of training group data, whereas only 36% of those for the successful group were in this category. Centrative perceptual activity was also more apparent in the unsuccessful group than in the successful group. Here the data indicated that 55% of the relevant observations of unsuccessful children showed centrative perceptual activity, but only 37% of the observations of successful children. In addition, successful subjects showed a greater percentage of verbal responses attributing apparent conservation violations to legerdemain (87% vs. 57%) and a greater percentage of surprise reactions than unsuccessful subjects (56% vs. 33%). It would therefore appear that the eye-movement and surprise reaction data of subjects for whom training was effective was even more closely comparable with that of natural conservers than the analyses of training group data might have originally suggested. At the same time, since the amount of experience involved in training is probably considerably less than is encountered during natural conservation acquisition, it does not seem surprising that differences between trained conservers and nonconservers are somewhat less striking than natural conserver-nonconserver differences.

The results of this study seem to have at least one clear implication for

46

Piaget's (1947, 1970) theoretical position. Specifically, it would appear that in terms of cognitive structural changes the development of intelligence as evidenced by the acquisition of conservation can be accelerated to a substantial degree in normal children.

STUDY 3. PERCEPTUAL ACTIVITY AND SURPRISE REACTIONS IN MILDLY RETARDED CONSERVERS AND NONCONSERVERS

Results

Retarded conservers were generally slower than retarded nonconservers in reaching task decisions. Analysis of eye-movement data in terms of a common time interval thus seemed necessary, and the first three seconds of decision period were again used for this purpose.

Conservation tasks. The following results of between group analyses of general perceptual activity involved the use of a Groups (conservers vs. nonconservers) by Tasks (I and II) analysis of variance with repeated measures on Tasks. Conservers, in comparison with nonconservers, showed more runs ($\bar{X}_{rc} = 2.40$, $\bar{X}_{rnc} = 1.70$; $F = 11.594$, $df = 1/28$, $p < .01$).* more fixations ($\bar{X}_{rc} = 12.00$, $\bar{X}_{rnc} = 8.20$; $F = 27.814$, $df = 1/28$, $p < .001$), and a shorter mean length of fixation in one tenth second units, over both elements ($\bar{X}_{rc} = 2.69$, $\bar{X}_{rnc} = 3.73$; $F = 18.953$, $df = 1/28$, $p < .001$). In addition, both groups showed more fixations on Task I ($\bar{X}_{I} = 10.80$, $\bar{X}_{II} = 9.40$; $F = 10.559$, $df = 1/28$, $p < .01$). All other main and interaction effects were nonsignificant. These results provide some support for Hypothesis 3.1 indicating, as with normal subjects, that there were also differences between retarded conservers and nonconservers in terms of general perceptual activity. It should be pointed out, however, that these findings were not as strong as those reported for normal subjects, specifically since significant couplings and mean length of run effects were not observed.

Table 3 presents mean values for Tasks I and II (calculated as in Studies 1 and 2) and correlated *t* test data. These within group analyses reveal that on the greater element nonconservers had more runs ($t = 3.14$, $df = 14$, $p < .01$), a greater mean length of run ($t = 3.53$, $df = 14$,

* Lower case letters rc and rnc are used to refer, respectively, to retarded conservers and retarded nonconservers.

47

$p < .01$), more fixations ($t = 3.60$, $df = 14$, $p < .01$), a greater mean length of fixation ($t = 3.28$, $df = 14$, $p < .01$) and more examination time in tenths of seconds ($t = 3.82$, $df = 14$, $p < .001$). At the same time conservers showed a greater frequency of runs ($t = 2.38$, $df = 14$, $p < .05$) and more examination time on the transformed element ($t = 2.08$, $df = 14$, $p < .05$). All other interelement differences were nonsignificant. Consequently, Hypotheses 3.2 and 3.3 received some support. Specifically, it appears that centrative perceptual activity differentiates retarded conservers and nonconservers, although not to the extent it did with normal subjects where conservers showed no interelement differences on frequency of runs and amount of examination time.

Table 3. Summary of correlated t tests on Tasks I and II eye-movement data for retarded subjects

	Nonconservers			Trained Conservers			Conservers		
	GE$\overline{X}$[a]	LE$\overline{X}$[b]	t	TE$\overline{X}$[c]	NTE$\overline{X}$[d]	t	TE$\overline{X}$	NTE$\overline{X}$	t
Number of runs	1.73	0.93	3.14**	1.80	1.68	0.53	2.10	1.50	2.38**
Mean length of run	20.06	8.91	3.53**	16.70	11.76	1.77*	17.20	12.63	1.49
Number of fixations	8.07	4.68	3.60**	9.35	8.08	1.13	10.27	7.98	1.63
Mean length of fixation	5.50	3.93	3.28**	4.59	3.15	5.06***	3.70	3.30	1.15
Amount of examination time	24.00	10.25	3.82***	21.07	15.50	1.97*	22.95	15.60	2.08*

[a]GE$\overline{X}$ Mean value on element chosen as greater
[b]LE$\overline{X}$ Mean value on element chosen as lesser
[c]TE$\overline{X}$ Mean value on transformed element
[d]NTE$\overline{X}$ Mean value on nontransformed element
* $p < .05$
** $p < .01$
*** $p < .001$

Violation tasks. The apparent violations of conservation were attributed to legerdemain by significantly more conservers than nonconservers (97% vs. 20%; $z = 5.70$, $p < .0001$). Surprise reactions also differentiated the groups (Conservers 40% vs. Nonconservers 13%; $z = 2.34$, $p < .01$). Thus Hypothesis 3.4 was supported. Therefore, as in Studies 1 and 2, the occurrence of surprise reactions seems to reflect conservation violation recognition.

48

Table 4 summarizes within group analyses of Task III centrative perceptual activity. Comparisons between elements for conservers revealed that these subjects had more runs ($t = 3.60$, $df = 14$, $p < .01$), a greater mean length of run ($t = 2.49$, $df = 14$, $p < .05$), more fixations ($t = 3.27$, $df = 14$, $p < .01$) and spent more examination time ($t = 3.46$, $df = 14$, $p < .01$), on the transformed element. This table also shows that nonconservers made more runs on the transformed element ($t = 2.30$, $df = 14$, $p < .05$) and had a significantly longer mean length of fixation in one tenth second units on the transformed element ($t = 1.79$, $df = 14$, $p < .05$). None of the remaining interelement differences were significant for either group. Hypothesis 3.5 therefore received some support.

More specifically, for conservers, four of the five interelement differences in Table 4 were significant whereas only two were significant in Table 3. Increase in the transformed-nontransformed element ratio were observed on mean length of run and frequency of fixations on the part of conservers with the greatest centration being associated with the transformed element. It is also interesting to note the large increase in amount of examination time on the transformed element over that observed on the greater element in Table 3. Nonconservers, on the other hand, showed fewer significant interelement differences in Table 4, although largest values were always associated with the transformed element. Similar findings were reported for normal nonconservers in Study 1. These findings suggest that conserver-nonconserver differences in retarded subjects are consistent with, but not as strong as those observed in normals.

Table 4. Summary of correlated t tests on Task III eye movement data for retarded subjects

	Nonconservers			Trained Conservers			Conservers		
	$_{TE}\overline{X}^a$	$_{NTE}\overline{X}^b$	t	$_{TE}\overline{X}$	$_{NTE}\overline{X}$	t	$_{TE}\overline{X}$	$_{NTE}\overline{X}$	t
Number of runs	1.53	1.10	2.30*	1.73	1.43	0.92	2.07	0.97	3.60**
Mean length of run	20.71	12.62	1.35	19.30	11.63	1.51	21.29	9.08	2.49*
Number of fixations	8.40	5.53	1.75	9.30	6.17	1.51	13.13	6.83	3.27**
Mean length of fixation	4.62	3.09	1.79*	4.34	3.57	1.51	3.38	2.60	1.27
Amount of examination time	23.63	14.20	1.71	23.40	14.50	1.67	28.03	11.30	3.46**

$^a_{TE}\overline{X}$	Mean value on transformed element
$^b_{NTE}\overline{X}$	Mean value on nontransformed element
*	$p < .05$
**	$p < .01$

In summary, retarded conservers, in comparison with retarded non-conservers, showed a number of predicted differences in general and centrative perceptual activity on conservation tasks (Tasks I and II). Predicted intergroup differences were also obtained for verbal responses and surprise reactions to conservation violations (Task III), and in retarded conservers, a predicted change in centrative perceptual activity occurred during violation tasks.

Discussion

The hypotheses which related to intergroup differences in general and centrative perceptual activity received considerable support from between and within group analyses of Task I and II eye-movement data. General perceptual behavior of retarded conservers was considerably more active than that shown by retarded nonconservers. A clear tendency for non-conservers to center more often and for longer periods on the element judged to be greater following transformation was also apparent, however, this trend was not strongly noticeable for conservers.

Verbal and surprise reactions to apparent violations of conservation also differentiated the groups in the predicted direction. The intergroup verbal response differences were in agreement with the contention that the transformation outcome expectancies of conservers and nonconservers prior to transformation completion were very different. Furthermore, it seems highly likely that the intergroup surprise reaction differences which were obtained arose from the fact that a greater percentage of these expectancies were violated for conservers.

Some support was also obtained for the hypothesis that nonconservers would show similar centrative perceptual activity on violation tasks, whereas conservers would show greater centrative behavior on Task III, than on Tasks I and II. The predicted centrative effect is probably best observed on the examination time variable, where a doubling in the ratio score difference in terms of more time being spent on the transformed element as opposed to the greater element, was observed. Thus, the data of Study 3 suggested the presence of differential cognitive functioning in retarded conservers and nonconservers.

Study 1 (normals) and the present study seem to have resulted in the documentation of a number of similar conserver – nonconserver differences which presumably reflect different levels of cognitive structural development. For example, similar patterns of conserver – nonconserver verbal response differences were obtained from both normal and retarded subjects. Likewise, perceptual activity and surprise reactions from normal and retarded subjects clearly differentiated conservers from nonconservers. At the same time, while similar conserver-nonconserver perceptual activity differences were observed in normal and retarded subjects, they were not as strong in retardates. Specifically, frequency of couplings and mean length of run, which clearly differentiated the general perceptual activity of normal conservers and nonconservers, and frequency of runs and time on the transformed element, which clearly differentiated the centrative perceptual activity of normal conservers and nonconservers, did not differentiate retarded conservers and nonconservers, did not differentiate retarded conservers and nonconservers. Conserver – nonconserver differences in eye-movement activity during conservation violation tasks were also not equivalent in normal and retarded subjects. Whereas normal conservers showed marked changes in all measures of centrative perceptual activity during Task III, a similar change was observed on only two of these dependent variables with retarded conservers.

The inconsistencies in general and centrative perceptual activity results discussed above may be due to a number of factors. They could be attributable to the fact that retarded subjects were considerably older than the normals, and this may have tended to reduce conserver-nonconserver general and centrative perceptual activity differences. Another possibility is that the above mentioned inconsistencies were reflecting an underlying normal-retardate attention differential of the type postulated by Zeaman and House (1963) and O'Connor and Hermelin (1963). A more interesting supposition would be that the cognitive structural development of the retarded conservers had not reached a level equivalent to that shown by the normals. Such a supposition would be in accord with Inhelder's (1963) suggestion that the closure of an operational system in mentally retarded children is of a different type from that found in normal children. Since all of the above possibilities are tenable, further research in this area is clearly necessary. It is interesting to note, however, that the findings of the present studies generally seem supportive of the notion of attentional and operational differences in retarded and normal children.

STUDY 4. PERCEPTUAL ACTIVITY AND SURPRISE REACTIONS IN TRAINED MILDLY RETARDED CONSERVERS AND MILDLY RETARDED NONCONSERVERS

Results

Conservation tasks: verbal data. Analyses of immediate posttest data indicated distinct intergroup differences. Trained retarded conservers, in comparison with retarded nonconservers, showed a significantly higher proportion of logical conservation responses on Task I (100% vs. 0%; $z = 7.81$, $p < .0001$) and Task II (57% vs. 0%; $z = 4.89$, $p < .0001$). Similar group differences were also apparent for three week retention tests (Task I: 96% vs. 10%, $z = 6.71$, $p < .0001$; Task II: 80% vs. 6%, $z = 5.78$, $p < .0001$). The above results indicate that the training procedure was successful with mentally retarded children in terms of generalizability and relative permanence of verbal data.

Conservation tasks: eye-movement data. Trained retarded nonconservers tended to take longer to reach task decisions than retarded nonconservers. Analysis of eye-movement data in terms of a constant time interval (first three seconds) was therefore undertaken as in Studies 1, 2, and 3.

Between group analyses of Task I and II general perceptual activity data were conducted, as in previous studies, using a Groups (trained retarded conservers and retarded nonconservers) by Tasks (I & II) analysis of variance design with repeated measures on Tasks. The following results were obtained. In comparison with retarded nonconservers, trained retarded conservers showed, summed over both elements, more runs ($\bar{X}_{rt} = 2.20$, $\bar{X}_{rnc} = 1.70$; $F = 4.805$, $df = 1/28$, p $< .05$),* more fixations ($\bar{X}_{rt} = 11.24$, $\bar{X}_{rnc} = 2.80$; $F = 11.336$, $df = 1/28$, $p < .01$), and a shorter mean length of fixation in one tenth second units ($\bar{X}_{rt} = 2.95$, $\bar{X}_{rnc} = 3.73$; $F = 7.205$, $df = 1/28$, $p < .05$). Both groups showed on Task I, summed over both elements, more runs ($\bar{X}_I = 2.25$, $\bar{X}_{II} = 1.65$; $F = 18.705$, $df = 1/28$, $p < .0001$), more fixations ($\bar{X}_I = 10.75$, $\bar{X}_{II} = 8.69$; $F = 17.394$, $df = 1/28$, $p < .0001$), and a shorter mean length of fixation ($\bar{X}_I = 3.00$, $\bar{X}_{II} = 3.68$; $F = 11.901$, $df = 1/28$, $p < .01$). All remaining analyses of general perceptual activity in terms of main and interaction effects were nonsignificant. These results although not as strong as those reported in Study 2, do provide support for Hypothesis 4.1. Moreover, they indicate in mildly retarded children, differential general perceptual activity on the part of trained conservers and nonconservers.

Within group analyses of Task I and II centrative perceptual activity were undertaken using correlated t tests. Table 3 presents the results of these analyses. Nonconservers showed more runs ($t = 3.14$, $df = 14$, $p < .01$), a greater mean length of run ($t = 3.53$, $df = 14$, $p < .01$), more fixations ($t = 3.60$, $df = 14$, $p < .01$), a greater mean length of fixation

---

* Lower case letters rt and rnc are used to refer, respectively, to trained retarded conservers and retarded nonconservers.

($t = 3.28$, $df = 14$, $p < .01$) and a greater amount of examination time ($t = 3.82$, $df = 14$, $p < .001$) on the greater element. Trained conservers, on the other hand, showed a greater mean length of run ($t = 1.77$, $df = 14$, $p < .05$), a greater mean length of fixation ($t = 5.06$, $df = 14$, $p < .001$), and spent a greater amount of examination time on the transformed element ($t = 1.97$, $df = 14$, $p < .05$). All other differences were nonsignificant. Some support was thus obtained for Hypothesis 4.2, but not as much as for Hypothesis 4.3. In line with this, it should also be noted, that Hypothesis 4.2., which states that trained conservers will show minimum centrative perceptual activity, was less strongly supported than an equivalent one in Study 3 with natural conservers. Consequently, findings associated with this hypothesis should be interpreted with some caution.

Violation tasks. Trained retarded conservers and retarded nonconservers were differentiated on the basis of their verbal responses to conservation violation items. Whereas 73% of trained conservers attributed the apparent conservation violations to legerdemain, only 20% of the nonconservers responded in this way ($z = 4.34$, $p < .0001$). A similar trend was obtained with surprise reactions where a significantly greater percentage of surprise reactions were shown by trained retarded conservers than nonconservers following conservation violations (36% vs. 13%, $z = 2.09$, $p < .025$). Hypothesis 4.4 was therefore supported and as in Studies 1, 2, and 3, the occurrence of surprise reactions appears to reflect conservation violation recognition.

Within group analyses of Task III centrative perceptual activity were also undertaken and are reported in Table 4. Nonconservers showed with respect to the transformed and nontransformed elements more runs ($t = 2.30$, $df = 14$, $p < .01$) and a greater mean length of fixation ($t = 1.79$, $df = 14$, $p < .05$) on the transformed element. While these results are not in agreement with those obtained from similar analyses of Task I and II data (Table 3), they are nevertheless consistent to the extent that the largest values are always associated with the transformed element. Task I and II analyses for nonconservers also resulted in significant inter-element differences in favor of the greater element on all dependent variables. On Task III two of these differences were still significant, two were marginally significant, and, on the remaining dependent variable the mean for the transformed element was higher than that for the nontransformed element. None of the interelement differences were significant for trained conservers. Thus, the results do not generally provide strong support for Hypothesis 4.5, especially since the perceptual activity of trained conservers did not appear to increase on the transformed element as a function of the conservation violations.

In summary, trained retarded conservers, in comparison with retarded nonconservers, showed a number of predicted differences in general and centrative perceptual activity on conservation tasks (Tasks I and II). Predicted intergroup differences in verbal responses and surprise reactions to conservation violations (Task III) were also obtained, but predicted changes in centrative perceptual activity on the part of trained nonconservers were not.

Discussion

The between and within group analyses of Task I and II eye-movement data clearly differentiated trained retarded conservers and retarded nonconservers and provided support for the experimental hypotheses. Specifically, it was found in terms of corneally reflected eye movements, that trained conservers showed more general perceptual activity than nonconservers, and that nonconservers centered more often, and for longer periods, on the element judged to be greater following transformation. Therefore, general and centrative perceptual activity during Tasks I and II, in addition to verbal response data, appear to offer support for the contention that the conservation acceleration procedure had successfully induced a degree of cognitive structural change. This change, however, appeared to be not as great as it had been with normal subjects in Study 2.

Analyses of verbal and surprise reaction data during conservation violation tasks also yielded predicted intergroup differences. These results suggest that pretransformation expectancies with respect to the transformation outcome were very different in trained conservers and nonconservers. Indeed, it would appear that prior to the transformations more trained conservers than nonconservers had expected that quantity or length would remain invariant despite stimulus transformation. The fact that the transformation outcome was violated seems likely to have led to the intergroup surprise reaction differences which were obtained. The hypothesis associated with an increase in centrative perceptual activity on the part of trained conservers during conservation violation tasks was not supported. While it might appear that the training procedure was slightly less effective with retarded than normal subjects, it should be recalled that retarded conservers (Study 3) showed centrative perceptual activity on Task III different from that of normal conservers (Study 1). This finding might suggest differential cognitive functioning in normal and retarded children.

Eye-movement data during conservation tasks and surprise reaction data during conservation violation tasks seem to strengthen the claim, which could be made on the basis of verbal response data, that the conservation acceleration procedure had been effective in inducing cognitive structural change in the mildly retarded training group. Thus, from the standpoint of Piaget's (1947, 1970) theoretical position, it would appear that the development of intelligence, as evidenced by the acquisition of conservation, can be accelerated to a substantial degree in preoperational mildly retarded children. Although the present study was concerned with only one aspect of intellectual development within Piaget's theory, the above result seems consistent with the findings of previous studies which have indicated that intellectual development in terms of intelligence test performance can be accelerated in mentally retarded children (e.g., Skeels & Dye, 1939; Kirk, 1958; Spicker, Hodges, & McCandless, 1966).

It is possible that the training effects could have been suppressed to some extent since the training was relatively ineffective for several subjects in the trained conserver group. While all of the trained conservers showed conservation responses on Task I (the task on which they were trained), only 57% showed conservation responses on Task II. It would therefore appear that a number of subjects were giving pseudoconservation responses as a function of training. The inclusion of data from these subjects in the analyses of training effects should have attenuated differences between trained conservers and nonconservers. Consequently, as in Study 2, a comparison was made of eye-movement, surprise reaction, and verbal response data on conservation violation tasks between the ten subjects for whom training had been successful (i.e., subjects who showed conservation responses on both Task I and II immediate posttests and three week retention tests) and the five subjects for whom training appeared to be unsuccessful.

While some support was provided for the above contention of a suppression effect, a degree of inconsistency was apparent. General perceptual behavior, as in Study 2, seemed less active in unsuccessful subjects. For the unsuccessful group, 68% of relevant observations were below the training group means used in the analyses of training group data (or in the case of duration of runs and fixations, were above the training group means), whereas only 37% of those for the successful group were in this category. Furthermore, successful subjects showed more verbal responses attributing apparent conservation violations to legerdemain (85% vs. 30%). Indications of centrative perceptual activity responses (51% vs. 55%) and percentage of surprise reactions (30% vs. 50%) for successful and unsuccessful subjects, respectively, however, did not differentiate the groups. Thus, the inclusion of data from unsuccessful subjects probably did not attenuate training effects for retarded subjects to any great extent.

This result is somewhat puzzling. It seems to suggest again that language and psychophysiological activity were differentially related in normal and retarded training groups. Such a possibility might arise, in part, because of different language and thinking processes in normals and retardates (Shif, 1969). It could also be a function of a basic retardate attention-orientation reaction deficit of the type postulated by Zeaman and House (1963) and Luria (1963), or it could reflect the fact that the retarded subjects were considerably older than the normals.

There is, however, another possibility. While there were five subjects who failed to show conservation on Task II immediate posttests, four of these subjects actually showed conservation on Task II, three weeks later.

This suggests that training may have had an effect on conservation development in these subjects, which was not apparent immediately after training but did become so, three weeks later. Consequently it is possibly somewhat misleading using immediate posttest performance of these subjects as indicative of a lack of training effect.

4. Conclusions

Table 5 summarizes the results of between and within group comparisons on conservation and violation tasks in terms of percentage of statistical tests supportive for specific hypotheses. Table 6 summarizes conservation response (posttraining and retention), verbal awareness, and surprise reaction data for the four studies. These tables, considered jointly, help to emphasize the basic findings of the research.

Table 5. Summary of support for specific hypotheses based on percentage of statistical tests confirmed

Hypothesis		Studies			
Number	*Description*	*1*	*2*	*3*	*4*
1.1, 2.1, 3.1, 4.1	Natural or trained conservers will show greater general perceptual activity than nonconservers during the solution of conservation tasks.	S[a]	S	G	G
1.2, 2.2, 3.2, 4.2	Natural or trained conservers will show minimum centrative perceptual activity during the solution of conservation tasks.	S	S	G	Q
1.3, 2.3, 3.3, 4.3	Nonconservers will show maximum centrative perceptual activity during the solution of conservation tasks.	S	S	S	S
1.4, 2.4, 3.4, 4.4	Natural or trained conservers in comparison with nonconservers will show more surprise reactions and verbal awareness of legerdemain following apparent violations of conservation.	S	S	S	S
1.4, 2.5, 3.5, 4.5	Nonconservers will show similar degrees of centrative perceptual activity during conservation and conservation violation task solution whereas natural or trained conservers will show an increase in centrative perceptual activity on violation tasks over that shown on conservation tasks.	G[b]	Q[c]	G	Q

[a]S   Strong support – 80% or more of comparisons confirmed
[b]G   General support – 50% – 79% of comparisons confirmed
[c]Q   Questionable support – less than 50% of comparisons confirmed

Table 6. Percentage of logical conservation and verbal awareness responses and surprise reactions for groups

Type of Response	Study 1		Study 2		Study 3		Study 4	
	nc	nnc	nt	nnc	rc	rnc	rt	rnc
Concervation (Posttraining)								
Task I			80	0[a]			100	0
Task II			47	0			57	0
Verbal Awareness	100	16	73	16	97	20	73	20
Surprise Reaction	53	17[b]	43	17	40	13	36	13[c]
Conservation (Retention)								
Task I			77	3			97	10
Task II			53	0			80	6

[a] All differences significant at $p < .001$ unless otherwise noted
[b] $p < .005$
[c] $p < .025$

Inspection of Table 5 with respect to normal and retarded natural conservers and nonconservers (Studies 1 and 3) indicates differential conserver-nonconserver general perceptual activity effects, with 100% (5/5) of the tests associated with Hypothesis 1.1 supportive and 60% (3/5) of those with Hypothesis 3.1. A comparison of centrative perceptual activity hypotheses also reveals conserver-nonconserver differences. Here 100% (5/5) of the tests based on Hypothesis 1.2 were confirmed, 60% (3/5) for Hypothesis 3.2, and 100% (5/5) for both Hypotheses 1.3 and 3.3. Thus, conserver-nonconserver differences in general and centrative perceptual activity were evident in normals and retardates, with effects being slightly less strong for retardates. Conservers, irrespective of group, seemed generally more active in exploring the elements than nonconservers. And, they did not fixate on the transformed or apparently greater element to the extent that was evident in nonconservers.

The analyses of verbal awareness responses and surprise reactions during violation tasks also resulted in comparable conserver-nonconserver differences in normal and retarded subjects, with 100% (2/2) of the tests positive for Hypotheses 1.4 and 3.4. Table 6 shows that normal and retarded conservers gave, respectively, 100% and 97% verbal awareness responses (noticed the trick), and 53% and 40% surprise reactions. Concomitantly, nonconservers gave similar responses in 20% or less of the cases for both normal and retardate groups. In terms of centrative perceptual activity, the analyses of eye movements during violation tasks also revealed conserver-nonconserver differences in both normal and retarded children. Here 70% (7/10) of the statistical comparisons associated with Hypothesis 1.5 were supportive, and 50% (4/8) of those with Hypothesis 3.5. Although the above conserver-nonconserver effects were noticeable, they again seemed somewhat stronger in normals than retardates.

The training procedure (Studies 2 and 4) appears have been equally effective for both groups, especially when evaluated in terms of percentage of conservation responses given on posttraining and three week retention testing (See Table 6). In fact, on posttraining testing retarded subjects had 100% transfer on Task I and 57% on Task II, whereas normals showed only 80% and 47% transfer. This differential was also apparent on retention tests where retardates showed 97% and 80% conservation responses on Task I and II, and normals, comparatively, 77% and 53% such responses. Differences between trained conserver and nonconserver groups for both normals and retardates were all statistically significant beyond the .001 level. Thus, there seems little doubt that the training procedure worked. At the same time the data reveals that training was not equally effective for all subjects, since about one-half of the children failed to give conservation responses on all posttraining and retention tests.

Results of eye-movement analyses indicate trained conserver-nonconserver differences, but again the data suggest slightly weaker effects for retardates (See Table 5). For example, whereas there were noticeable differences in general perceptual activity for both groups, 100% (5/5) of the tests for Hypothesis 2.1 were positive, but only 60% (3/5) of those for Hypothesis 4.1. Centrative perceptual activity analyses also suggest slight normal-retarded differences, particularly in terms of the hypothesis predicting minimum centrative activity for trained conservers. Here 100% (5/5) of the tests associated with Hypothesis 2.2 were significant, but only 40% (2/5) of those for Hypothesis 4.2. On the other hand, strong centrative effects were observed for both groups of nonconservers with 100% (5/5) of the tests associated with Hypotheses 2.3 and 4.3 supportive. The above data suggests that the preoperational behavior of normal and retarded children was somewhat similar. And that the perceptual activity of trained conservers was generally much like that of natural conservers.

Verbal awareness and surprise reaction responses also differentiated trained conserver from nonconserver groups with 100% (2/2) of the tests associated with Hypotheses 2.4 and 4.4 confirmed. Table 6 shows that trained normal and retarded conserver groups gave the same percentage of verbal awareness responses (73%) and, respectively, 43% and 36% surprise reactions. Correspondingly, nonconservers gave similar responses in 20% or less of the cases. Normal and retarded trained conservers, in comparison with nonconservers, however, did not show predicted changes in centrative perceptual activity during the violation tasks. In fact, only 30% (3/10) and 20% (2/10), respectively, of the tests associated with Hypotheses 2.5 and 4.5 were in the predicted direction. In contrast, natural normal conservers, and to a lesser extent, retarded conservers showed predicted changes.

Overall, it might appear that the training procedure was slightly less effective with retarded than normal children. This possibility can be somewhat discounted, however, since for both normal and retarded subjects the performance data of the training groups closely approximated that shown by their respective natural conserver groups. The apparent normal-retardate training differences may also have been reduced if, as previously mentioned, analyses had been conducted only on those subjects who gave conservation responses on all posttraining and retention tests. Yet, a comparison of Studies 1 and 2, with Studies 3 and 4 (Table 5), reveals eight strongly supported hypotheses for normals, but only four for retardates. This table also shows two changes in overall support of hypotheses in Study 4 in comparison with Study 3, but only one change between Studies 1 and 2. Consequently, it appears that there is differential cognitive functioning (eye-movement activity) in retarded and normal children at these age levels. Moreover, these differences seem apparent in both natural conserver and trained conserver groups.

Several additional eye-movement studies, using retarded children of about the same age, IQ, and background characteristics as those used in the present investigation also deserve mention. These studies also suggest the possibility of differential cognitive activity in retardates as reflected by eye-movement behavior. Concomitantly, it should be noted that in the following studies, unlike the present one, attempts were made to match normal and retarded subjects on chronological age.

In one of these, Boersma and Muir (in preparation) presented 24 normals ($\bar{X}_{age} = 126.8_{mos.}$; $\bar{X}_{IQ} = 113.0$) and 20 retardates ($\bar{X}_{age} = 125.3_{mos.}$; $\bar{X}_{IQ} = 72.4$) with a two-choice discrimination learning task. The stimuli contained three basic discriminable dimensions (position, form and number) with the relevant dimension being number (of dots) and the appropriate cue odd (1 or 3). Two verbal instructional treatments were also presented, one after trial 10 and the other after trial 20. In Treatment 1 the subjects were instructed to look at the dots, whereas in Treatment 2 they were provided with the actual mediational link, i.e., the solution to the problem. Treatment effects were evident for normals, but not for retardates. Moreover, retarded children showed distinct evidence of attentional difficulties, irrespective of whether they learned or not. Specifically, their eye-movement activity indicated an

60

inability to focus on relevant information (fewer frames on relevant cues and more unscoreable data) even when instructed as to what to look at. But, perhaps even more interesting from the perspective of the present series of studies, was the suggestion in the data of a retardate developmental lag in appropriate looking behavior, and the indication that visual search of retarded learners was less efficient (apparently) than that of normal learners. Thus, these data also indicate the possibility of differential cognitive functioning (eye-movement activity) in normal and retarded children.

Two pictorial visual search studies provide further support for the supposition of eye movement differences during cognitive problem solving in normal and retarded children. For example, Muir and Boersma (in preparation) presented the same subjects used in the discrimination learning study with two sets of pictorial stimuli. The first set consisted of three pictures, each containing an inappropriate aspect in the stimulus complex and subjects were asked to locate what was wrong with the picture. The second set of three pictures showed some event occurring and the children were asked to tell what was happening in the picture. Informative search scores, of the type discussed by Conklin, Muir and Boersma (1968), were significantly lower for retarded children on both tasks, thus indicating that retardates spent less time focusing on highly informative areas than did normals, despite similar chronological ages. The data also indicated, although somewhat less strongly this time, that the mean duration of fixation for retardates was shorter than that for normals. Mackworth and Bruner (1970) have reported visual search differences between normal adults and normal children, with adults having higher informative search scores. Their primary emphasis was on developmental differences as a function of age, although they also considered the possibility of cognitive development affecting eye-movement behavior. The above results, considered jointly with those of O'Bryan and Boersma (1971) and the present series of studies, indicate that eye-movement differences are indeed related to cognitive (mental) development

The second. study investigated initial and habituated visual search in normal and retarded children, in comparison with a group of undergraduate college students (Boersma, Barham, & Rogers, in preparation). Ninety subjects were tested, 30 in each of 3 groups, with each subject being exposed to 5 pictures for a period of 60 seconds. These pictures were fairly complex showing the occurrence of an event and of high interest value. Mean ages in months and WISC characteristics for the samples were as follows (College: $\bar{X}_{age} = 285.2$; Normal: $\bar{X}_{age} = 136.0$,

$\bar{X}_{IQ} = 118.8$; Retarded: $\bar{X}_{age} = 131.5$, $\bar{X}_{IQ} = 70.4$). The data were scored in terms of informative search scores and unscorable frames for the first and last five seconds of exposure. In 100% of the cases college students had higher mean search scores than normals, and in 90% of the comparisons normals had higher mean scores than retardates. Moreover, there was pronounced visual search habituation for all groups, with the effect being most noticeable for retardates. Analyses of unscorable frames also revealed group differences. Here, retardates had more unscorable data than normals and college students, and again the effect was most obvious for them during habituation trials. Thus, the data suggest that efficiency of visual search relative to pictorial material increases with age and/or mental development, and more specifically, that eye-movement behavior of retarded children is different, at least somewhat so, from normal children of equivalent age.

Inhelder (1963) has suggested that retarded subjects do not proceed beyond the level of concrete operations and that their structural development tends to be characterized by a closure of operational structures which differs from that shown by normals. Perhaps this is what the above discussed studies reflect. The results of Studies 1–2, and 3–4, certainly seem consistent with her position. In addition, the close similarity of retardate and normal verbal response data, together with the inconsistencies between the groups noted in eye-movement and surprise reaction data, might also indicate that language and thinking are differentially related in normal and retarded children, as suggested by Shif (1969).

Finally, it should be pointed out that normal-retarded developmental comparisons are extremely difficult to interpret since obtained differences could be a function of a number of uncontrollable factors. For example, there are wide differences between normals and retardates with respect to ages at which Piagetian stages are reached (Inhelder, 1963; Woodward, 1963). Moreover, differences between normal and retarded groups in terms of mental ages, learning histories, motivational factors, etc., are also likely at comparable developmental levels. Any or all of these variables could contribute substantially to intergroup differences. Yet, the present series of studies, considered jointly with the previously mentioned discrimination learning and visual search studies, indicates that eye-movement behavior of normals and retardates is indeed different. Perhaps this reflects the lack of co-ordination between analysis and synthesis in the retarded children.

In closing, several comments should be made about the training part of the current series of studies. The procedure seems to have been effective in accelerating conservation acquisition, and it would thus appear that conservation acquisition is one aspect of intellectual development which can be accelerated in preoperational normal and mentally retarded children. The data of the present studies, however, indicate that it may be slightly more difficult to do so with retardates.

The significance of conservation acceleration in a more molar sense, however, is not yet clear. According to Piaget (1947, 1970) conservation acquisition is a critical step in intellectual development, therefore, it seems likely that the successful inducement of conservation would have a substantial influence on subsequent cognitive functioning. While the present study was not concerned with this relationship, a logical next step would be to examine the effects of accelerated conservation acquisition on other areas of cognitive functioning. It may well be that induced conservation acquisition needs to be accompanied by accelerated acquisition of a number of other aspects of concrete operational functioning before the influence on cognitive activity in general becomes apparent.

At the same time the training results may not reflect conservation acquisition *de novo*, but rather successful communication to the subject of the exact behavior required for the task which may have been in his repertoire before training was undertaken (Gelman, 1969). It is obviously important to examine the above possibility in some detail. If in fact the above is found to be the case, the influence of the induced conservation acquisition on other aspects of cognitive functioning would probably be minimal. However, to the extent that conservation task performance defines conservation status, the present results may be interpreted as an acceleration of conservation acquisition. Moreover, in view of the substantial differences between trained conservers and nonconservers, and the striking similarities between these differences and those observed between natural conservers and nonconservers, it seems likely that the effects of training in the present series of studies were by no means slight.

References

Achenbach, T.M., Conservation of illusion-distorted identity: Its relation to MA and CA in normals and retardates. *Child Development*, 1969, *40*, 663–679.

Achenbach, T.M., Surprise and GSR as indicators of conservation: A new approach to developmental diagnosis demonstrated with retardates. *Proceedings, 78th Annual Convention*, APA, 1970, *78*, 281–282.

Beilin, H., The training and acquisition of logical operations. In M.S. Rosskopf, L.P. Steffe, & S. Taback (Eds.), *Piagetetian cognitive-development research and mathematical education*. Washington: National Council of Teachers of Mathematics, 1971. Pp. 81–124.

Berlyne, D.E., *Conflict, arousal and curiosity*. New York: McGraw-Hill, 1960.

Berlyne, D.E., Motivational problems raised by exploratory and epistemic behavior. In S. Koch (Ed.), *Psychology: A study of a science*, Vol. 5, New York, McGraw-Hill, 1963, 284–364.

Berlyne, D.E., *Structure and direction in thinking*. New York: Wiley, 1965.

Berlyne, D.E., Attention as a problem in behavior theory. In D. Mostofsky (Ed.), *Attention: Contemporary theory and analysis*. New York: Appleton-Century-Crofts, 1970, Pp. 25–49.

Binet, A., *Les idees modernes sur les enfants*. Paris: Ernest Flamarion, 1909.

Blishen, B.R., The construction and use of an occupational class scale, *Canadian Journal of Economics and Political Science*, 1958, *24*, 519–531.

Boersma, F.J., & Muir, W., Visual searching behavior in normal and retarded children during discrimination learning, in preparation.

Boersma, F.J., Barham, R., & Rogers, T., Initial and habituated visual search in normal and retarded children and adults, in preparation.

Boersma, F.J., Muir, W., Wilton, K., & Barham, R., Eye movements during embedded figure tasks. *Perceptual and Motor Skills*, 1969, *28*, 271–274.

Boersma, F.J., Wilton, K., Barham, R., & Muir, W., Effects of arithmetic problem difficulty on pupillary dilation in normals and educable retardates. *Journal of Experimental Child Psychology*, 1970, *9*, 142–155.

Braine, M.D.S., The ontogeny of certain logical operations: Piaget's formulation examined by nonverbal methods. *Psychological Monographs*, 1959, *73*, (Whole No. 475).

Brainerd, C.J., & Allen, T.W., Experimental inductions of the conservation of 'first-order' quantitative invariants, *Psychological Bulletin*, 1971, *75*, 128–144.

Brison, D.W., & Bereiter, C., Acquisition of conservation of substance in normal, retarded and gifted children. In D.W. Brison & E.V. Sullivan (Eds.), *Recent research on the acquisition of conservation of substance*. Toronto: Ontario Institute for Studies in Education, 1967. Pp. 53–72.

Bruner, J.S., On cognitive growth. In J.S. Bruner et al.; *Studies in cognitive growth.* New York: Wiley, 1966. Pp. 1–67.

Campbell, D.T., & Stanley, J.C., *Experimental and quasi-experimental designs for research.* Chicago: Rand McNally, 1963.

Charlesworth, W.R., The growth of knowledge of the effects of rotation and shaking on the linear order of objects (Unpublished doctoral dissertation, Cornell University), New York, 1962.

Charlesworth, W.R., Instigation and maintenance of curiosity behavior as a function of surprise versus novel and familiar stimuli. *Child Development*, 1964, *35*, 1169–1186.

Charlesworth, W.R., Persistence of orienting and attending behavior in infants as a function of stimulus locus uncertainty. *Child Development*, 1966, *37*, 473–491.

Charlesworth, W.R., The role of surprise in cognitive development. In D. Elkind and J.H. Flavell (Eds.), *Studies in cognitive development: Essays in honor of Jean Piaget.* New York: Oxford University Press, 1969. Pp. 257–314.

Conklin, R.C., Muir, W., & Boersma, F.J., Field dependency-independency and eye-movement patterns. *Perceptual and Motor Skills*, 1968, *26*, 59–65.

Creelman, M.B., *The experimental investigation of meaning*, New York: Springer, 1966.

Crosby, K.G., & Blatt, B., Attention and mental retardation. *Journal of Education*, 1968, *150*, 67–81.

Doll, E. A., The essentials of an inclusive concept of mental deficiency. *American Journal of Mental Deficiency*, 1941, *46*, 214–219.

Elkind, D., Piagetian and psychometric conceptions of intelligence. *Harvard Educational Review*, 1969, *39*, 319–337.

Ferguson, G.A., *Statistical analysis in psychology and education* (2nd ed.). New York: McGraw-Hill, 1966.

Flavell, J.H., *The developmental psychology of Jean Piaget*. Princeton, New Jersey: Van Nostrand, 1963.

Flavell, J.H., & Hill, J.P., Developmental psychology. In P. Mussen & M. Rosenzweig (Eds.), *Annual Review of Psychology*, 1969, *20*, 1–56.

Furth, H.G., *Thinking without language: Psychological implications of deafness*. New York: The Free Press, 1966.

Gelman, R., Conservation acquisition: A problem of learning to attend to relevant attributes. *Journal of Experimental Child Psychology*, 1969, *7*, 167–187.

Goddard, H.H., *The Kallikak family*, New York, MacMillan, 1912.

Graham, F., & Clifton, R., Heart-rate change as a component of the orienting response, *Psychological Bulletin*, 1966, *65*, 305–320.

Gray, J.A., Attention, consciousness and voluntary control of behavior in Soviet psychology: Philosophical roots and research branches. In N. O'Connor (Ed.), *Present day Russian psychology*. Oxford: Pergamon Press, 1966. Pp. 1–38.

Guskin, S.L., & Spicker, H.H., Educational research in mental retardation. In N.R. Ellis (Ed.). *International review of research in mental retardation*, Volume 3, New York, Academic Press, 1968. Pp. 217–278.

Hood, H.B., An experimental study of Piaget's theory of the development of number in children, *British Journal of Psychology*, 1962, *53*, 273–286.

Hunt, J. McV., *Intelligence and experience*, New York, Ronald Press, 1961.

Hunt, J. McV., Has compensatory education failed? Has it been attempted? *Harvard Educational Review*, 1969, *39*, 278–300.

Inhelder, B., Le diagnostic du raisonnement chez les débiles mentaux, (2nd ed.) Neuchatel: Delachaux & Niestle, 1963. (*The diagnosis of reasoning in the mentally retarded*, New York: John Day, 1968.)
Inhelder, B., Bovet M., Sinclair, H., & Smock, C.D., On cognitive development, *American Psychologist*, 1966, *21*, 160–164.
Itard, J.M.G., Rapports et memoires sur le sauvage de L'Averyon, Paris, 1806. (*The wild boy of Averyon*, New York: Appleton-Century-Crofts, 1932.)

Jeffery, W.E., The orienting reflex and attention in cognitive development. *Psychological Review*, 1968, *75*, 323–334.

Kingsley, R.C. & Hall, V.C., Conservation and equilibration theory. *Journal of Genetic Psychology*, 1968, *113*, 195–213.
Kirk, S.A., *Early education of the mentally retarded*. Urbana, Illinois: University of Illinois Press, 1958.
Kirk, S.A., Research in education. In R. Heber & H.A. Stevens (Eds.), *Mental retardation: A review of research*. Chicago: University of Chicago Press, 1964. Pp. 57–99.

Lewis, M., & Goldberg, S., The acquisition and violation of expectancy: An experimental paradigm. *Journal of Experimental Child Psychology*, 1969, *7*, 70–80.
Lewis, M., & Harwitz, M., The meaning of an orienting response: A study in the hierarchical order of attending, Paper presented at the meeting of the Society for Research in Child Development, Symposium on 'The Orienting Response: Issues in Developmental Inquiry', Santa Monica, California, March 1969.
Lister, C.M., The development of a concept of weight conservation in ESN children. *British Journal of Educational Psychology*, 1969, *39*, 245–252.
Lister, C.M., The development of a concept of volume conservation in ESN children. *British Journal of Educational Psychology*, 1970, *40*, 55–64.
Lister, C.M., The development of ESN children's understanding of conservation in a range of attribute situations. *British Journal of Educational Psychology*, 1972, *42*, 14–22.
Lord, F.M., Further problems in the measurement of growth. *Educational and psychological measurement*, 1958, *18*, 437–451.
Luria, A.R., *The mentally retarded child*. Oxford, Pergamon Press, 1963.
Lykken, D.T., Properties of electrodes used in electrodermal measurement. *Journal of Comparative and Physiological Psychology*, 1959, *52*, 629–634.
Lynn, R., *Attention, arousal and the orientation reaction*. Oxford: Pergamon Press, 1966.

Mackworth, N.H., A stand camera for line-of-sight recording. *Perception and Psychophysics*, 1967, *2*, 119–127.
Mackworth, N.H., & Bruner, J.S., How adults and children search and recognize pictures. *Human Development*, 1970, *13*, 149–177.
Maltzman, I., Individual differences in 'attention': The orienting reflex. In R. Gagné (Ed.), *Learning and individual differences*, Columbus, Ohio: Merrill, 1967. Pp. 94–112.
McNemar, Q., A critical examination of the University of Iowa studies of environmental influences upon the IQ. *Psychological Bulletin*, 1940, *37*, 63–92.

Mermelstein, E., & Meyer, E., Conservation training techniques and their effects on different populations. *Child Development*, 1969, *40*, 471–490.

Mermelstein, E., & Shulman, L.S., Lack of formal schooling and the acquisition of conservation. *Child Development*, 1967, *38*, 39–52.

Miller, S.A., Extinction of conservation: A methodological and theoretical analysis. *Merrill-Palmer Quarterly*, 1971, *17*, 319–334.

Montessori, M., *The Montessori method.* New York, Stokes, 1912.

Muir, W., & Boersma, F.J., Visual informative search in normal and retarded children, in preparation.

O'Bryan, K.G., & Boersma, F.J., Eye movements, perceptual activity and conservation, *Journal of Experimental Child Psychology*, 1971, *12*, 157–169.

O'Bryan, K.G., & Boersma, F.J., Movie presentation of Piagetian tasks: A procedure for the assessment of conservation attainment. *Journal of Genetic Psychology*, 1972, *121*, 295–302.

O'Connor, N., & Hermelin, B., *Speech and thought in severe subnormality.* Oxford, Pergamon Press, 1963.

Piaget, J., La psychologie de l'intelligence, Paris, Colin, 1947 (*The psychology of intelligence.* London: Routledge & Kegan Paul, 1950).

Piaget, J., Le problème neurologique de l'intériorisation des actions en opérations réversibles. *Archives de psychologie* (Genève), 1949, *32*, 241–258.

Piaget, J., Language and thought from the genetic point of view, *Acta Psychologica* 1954, *10*, 51–60. In D. Elkind (Ed.), Six études de psychologie, Geneva, Gonthier, 1964. (*Six psychological studies*, New York: Random House, 1967. Pp. 88–99.)

Piaget, J., Les stades du développement intellectuel de l'enfant et de l'adolescent. In P. Osterrieth et al., *Le problème des stades en psychologie de l'enfant*, Paris, Presses Universitaires de France, 1955, Pp. 33–113.

Piaget, J., (Problems of genetic psychology.), *Voprosy Psikhologii*, 1956. In D. Elkind (Ed.), Six études de psychologie, Geneva: Gonthier, 1964. *(Six psychological studies.* New York: Random House, 1967, Pp. 116–142.)

Piaget, J., The role of the concept and equilibrium in psychological explication. *Acta Psychologica*, 1959, *15*, 51–62. In D. Elkind (Ed.), *Six études de psychologie.* Geneva: Gauthier, 1964. (Six psychological studies. New York: Random House, 1967, Pp. 100–115.

Piaget, J., Les mécanismes perceptifs: modèles probabilistes, analyse génétique, relations avec l'intelligence. Paris: Presses Universitaires de France, 1961 (*The mechanisms of perception.* London: Routledge & Kegan Paul, 1969.)

Piaget, J., The stages of the intellectual development of the child, *Bulletin of the Menninger Clinic*, 1962, *26*, 120–128.

Piaget, J., The thought of the young child, Lecture given at the Institute of Education, University of London, 1963. In D. Elkind (Ed.), Six études de psychologie. Geneva: Gonthier, 1964. (*Six Psychological Studies.* New York: Random House, 1967, Pp. 77–86.) (a)

Piaget, J., Explanation in psychology and psychophysiological parallelism. In J. Piaget, P. Fraisse & M. Reuchlin (Eds.), Traité de psychologie expérimentale I: Histoire et méthode. Paris: Presses Universitaires de France, 1963. (*Experimental Psychology: Its scope and method.* London: Routledge & Kegan Paul, 1968, Pp. 153–191.) (b)

Piaget, J., Development and learning. In R.E. Ripple & V.N. Rockcastle (Eds.), *Piaget rediscovered: A report of the conference on cognitive studies and curriculum development.* Ithaca: School of Education, Cornell University, New York, 1964, Pp. 7–20 (a)

Piaget, J., The development of mental imagery. In R.E. Ripple & V.N. Rockcastle (Eds.), *Piaget rediscovered: A report of the conference on cognitive studies and curriculum development*. Ithaca: School of Education, Cornell University, New York, 1964, Pp. 21–39. (b)

Piaget, J., Review of J.S. Bruner, R.R. Olver, P.M. Greenfield, et al., Studies in cognitive growth. *Contemporary Psychology*, 1967, *12*, 532–533.

Piaget, J., Piaget's theory. In P.H. Mussen (Ed.), *Carmichael's manual of child psychology* (3rd ed.). New York: John Wiley and Sons, 1970, Pp. 703–732.

Piaget, J. & Inhelder, B., *Le développement des quantités physiques chez l'enfant: Conservation et atomisme*. (2nd ed.). Neuchatel: Delachaux et Niestle, 1962.

Piaget, J. & Inhelder, B., La psychologie de l'enfant, Collection 'Que sais-je' No. 369, Paris: Presses Universitaires de France, 1966. (*The psychology of the child*, New York, Basic Books, 1969.)

Piaget, J. & Szeminska, A., La genèse du nombre chez l'enfant. Neuchatel: Delachaux et Niestle, 1941. (*The child's conception of number*, New York, Humanities Press, 1952.)

Razran, G., The observable unconscious and the inferable conscious in current Soviet psychophysiology: Interoceptive conditioning, semantic conditioning, and the orienting reflex. *Psychological Review*, 1961, *68*, 81–147.

Reese, H.W. & Lipsitt, L.P., *Experimental child psychology*. New York, Academic Press, 1970.

Rosenthal, R., *Experimenter effects in behavioral research*. New York, Appleton-Century-Crofts, 1966.

Rosenthal, R., & Jacobsen, L., *Pygmalion in the classroom: Teacher expectation and pupils' intellectual development*. New York: Holt, Rinehart & Winston, 1968.

Schmalohr, E. & Winkelmann, W., Über den Einfluss der Übung auf die Entwicklung der Mengen und Substanzerhaltung beim Kinde, (On the influence of training with quality and substance conservation in children.). *Zeitschrift für Entwicklungspsychologie und Pädagogische Psychologie*, 1969, *2*, 93–102.

Seguin, E., *Idiocy, and its treatment by the physiological method*. Albany: New York, Brandow, 1866.

Shif, Z., Development of children in schools for the mentally retarded. In M. Cole & I. Maltzman (Eds.), *A handbook of contemporary Soviet psychology*. New York, Basic Books, 1969, Pp. 326–353.

Skeels, H.M., & Dye, H.B., A study of the effects of differential stimulation on mentally retarded children. *Journal of Psycho-Asthenics*, 1939, *44*, 114–136.

Smedlund, J., The acquisition of conservation of substance and weight in children. III. Extinction of conservation of weight acquired 'normally' and by means of empirical controls on a balance scale. *Scandinavian Journal of Psychology*, 1961, *2*, 85–87.

Sokolov, Ye, N., Vosprityatiye i uslovnyi refleks, Moscow, Moscow University Press, 1958. (*Perception and the conditioned reflex*, Oxford, Pergamon Press, 1963.)

Sokolov, Ye. N., Higher nerve functions: The orienting reflex. *Annual Review of Physiology*, 1963, *25*, 545–580.

Spicker, H.H., Hodges, W.L., & McCandless, B.R., A diagnostically based curriculum for psycho-socially deprived preschool mentally retarded children. *Exceptional Children*, 1966, *33*, 215–220.

Thorndike, R.L., Intellectual status and intellectual growth. *Journal of Educational Psychology*, 1966, *57*, 121–127.

Vygotsky, L.S., Myshlenie i rech'. Moscow: Academy of Pedagogical Sciences, 1956, (*Thought and language*. Cambridge, Massachusetts: MIT Press, 1962.)

Weinman, J., Photoplethysmography. In P.H. Venables & I. Martin (Eds.), *A manual of psychophysiological methods*. Amsterdam: North Holland Publishing Company, 1967, Pp. 185–218.

Winer, B.J., *Statistical principles in experimental design*, New York, McGraw-Hill, 1962.

Wohlwill, J., Piaget's theory of the development of intelligence in the concrete-operations period. In M. Garrison, Jr. (Ed.), *Cognitive models and development in mental retardation*, Monograph supplement to American Journal of Mental Deficiency, 1966, *70*, No. 4, Pp. 57–78.

Woodward, M., The application of Piaget's theory to research in mental deficiency. In N.R. Ellis (Ed.), *Handbook of mental deficiency*. New York: McGraw-Hill, 1963, 297–324.

Wright, J.C., Toward the assimilation of Piaget. *Merrill-Palmer Quarterly*, 1963, *9*, 277–285.

Zeaman, D., & House, B.J., The role of attention in retardate discrimination learning. In N.R. Ellis (Ed.), *Handbook of mental deficiency*. New York: McGraw-Hill, 1963, Pp. 159–223.